Entrepreneurship Development and Planning

Entrepreneurship Development and Planning

Manjeet Kalra
Astt. Professor
Dept. of Management and Humanities
Ajay Kumar Garg Engineering College, Ghaziabad

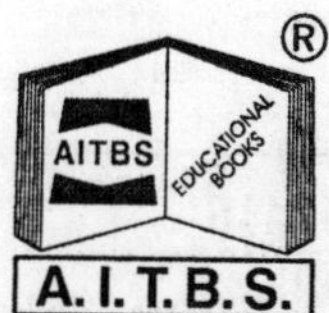

AITBS PUBLISHERS, INDIA
J-5/6, Krishan Nagar, Delhi-110051 (INDIA)
Tel.: 22054798, 22549313
Fax: 011-22543416
Email: aitbs@bol.net.in & aitbsindia@gmail.com

First Edition : 2008
Revised Reprint : 2012

ISBN: 978-81-7473-356-6

Published by:
Virender Kumar Arya for
AITBS Publishers, India
J-5/6, Krishan Nagar, Delhi-110051 (INDIA)
Phone: 22054798, 22549313; Fax: 011-22543416
E-mail: aitbs@bol.net.in & aitbsindia@gmail.com

Printed by AITBS, Delhi

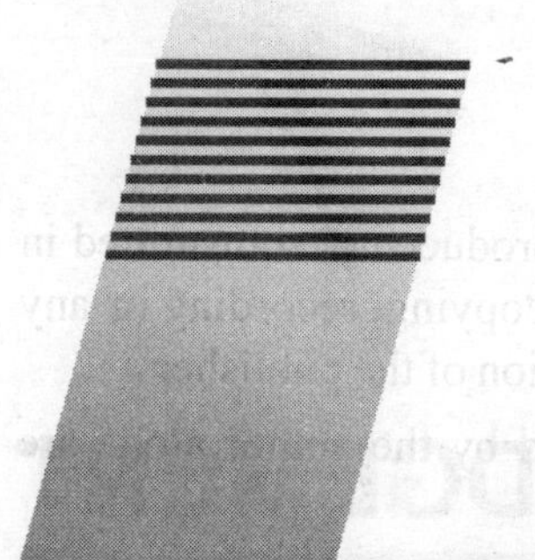

PREFACE

With the rapid industrialization and economic growth in the country there has been an enormous increase in the number and size of small scale industries. Small business serve as the seedbed of entrepreneurship.

If we go through the business history of India, we come across the name of many persons who have emerged as successful entrepreneurs. For example, Tata, Birla, Modi, Ambani, Narayanmurthy, etc. They all are well known names of successful entrepreneur who started their business entrepreneur with small size and good fortunes.

Entrepreneurship has now emerged as a profession. So much so that many entrepreneurship development institutes and centres have sprung up all over the country in recent years. Also many universities have already introduced Entrepreneurial Development as a subject in their graduate and post-graduate levels.

The present volume is a humble attempt to explain the various important aspects of the subject. This book analyses the start-up, development, support and management of small business and what a prospective entrepreneur must know before starting his own enterprise. Basic strength of this book are:

- Concise description of the subject
- Simple and conversational language
- Self-bearing style
- Universal application
- Student oriented
- Question bank

This book is of great help to students as well as to the teaching fraternity for a simple reason that they will find all relevant material related to the topic 'Entrepreneurship' in this one book. The comprehensive coverage ensures that all topics are found in this book.

I request colleagues in the teaching profession, students and all others who are interested in the study of entrepreneurship development to send their valuable and esteemed suggestions for the further improvement of this book. I am much obliged to Virender Kumar Arya of A.I.T.B.S. Publishers, India for being always extremely helpful and accommodoting.

Mrs. Manjeet Kalra

Astt. Professor

Dept. of Management

AKGEC, Ghaziabad

ACKNOWLEDGEMENT

A great many people have participated, directly or indirectly, in the preparation of this book. I would like to express my deep sense of gratitude to all of them.

No author can write in vaccum and I am certainly no exception. Vast reading of several books, websites and discussion with experts concerned enabled me to write this book. I am greatly indebted to all the authors (Specially Vasant Desai and Badai) and publishers of books on entrepreneurship and other related texts.

My family has played an important role in the completion of this book. I am appreciative and thankful to my husband Tanuj Kalra for his support, encouragement and help in the making of this book. And also my young son Keenan who provided a pleasurable source of distraction. I would be failing in my duty if I do not record my gratitude at a personal level to my parents Shri. B.L. Kalra and Smt. Chanderkanta Kalra and Shri Harbhajan Singh and Smt. Harjinder Kaur who brought me up to the present academic position.

I am beholden to Dr. R.K. Agarwal, Director, AKGEC, Gaziabad, whose encouragement has always shown us the right path.

I owe a special debt to my HOD, Prof. M.P. Dave, Dean Academics and HOD of Department of Electrical and Electronics and Applied Science and Management, AKGEC, Gaziabad for his guidance and encouragement.

This acknowledgment will not be complete without extending my sincerest thanks to the entire AKGEC, Gaziabad fraternity whose support and co-operation has always provided me with enthusiasm and Zeal to move forward.

Manjeet Kalra

SYLLABUS

OE-05 : Entrepreneurship Development Programme

(for Electronics, IT, C.S.), Elective Paper, VII Semester

Entrepreneur. Definition. Growth of small scale industries in developing countries and their positions vis-a-vis large industries; role of small scale industries in the national economy; characteristics and types of small scale industries; demand based and resources based ancillaries and sub-control type.

Government policy for small scale industry; stages in starting a small scale industry.

Project identification. Assessment of viability, formulation, evaluation, financing, field-study and collection of information, preparation of project report, demand analysis, material balance and output methods, benefit cost analysis, discounted cash flow, internal rate of return and net present value methods.

Accountancy. Preparation of balance sheets and assessment of economic viability, decision making, expected costs, planning and production control, quality control, marketing, industrial relations, sales and purchases, advertisement, wages and incentive, inventory control, preparation of financial reports, accounts and stores studies.

Project Planning and Control. The financial functions, cost of capital approach in project planning and control. Economic evaluation, risk analysis, capital expenditures, policies and practices in public enterprises, profit planning and programming, planning cash flow, capital expenditure and operations, control of financial flows, control and communication.

Laws concerning entrepreneur viz. partnership laws, business ownerships, sales and income taxes and workman compensation act.

Role of various national and state agencies which render assistance to small scale industries.

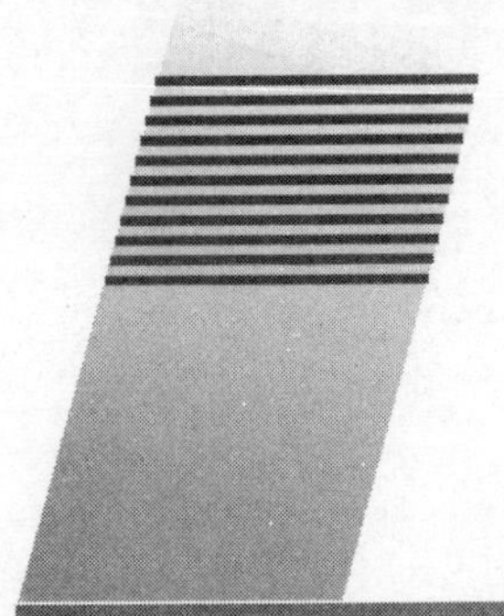

CONTENTS

1

The ...
means an ...

In the ...
expedition ...
the 17th ...
used to refer to ...
is considered ...

The ...
views are:

1. Entrepreneur ...

Richard ...
entrepreneur ...
century. ...
prices in ...
in future. ...

2. Entrepreneur ...

Jean Baptiste ...
function ...
entrepreneur ...
yet another ...
interest on ...
profit. ...

3. Entrepreneur ...

Joseph A. Schumpeter ...
entrepreneur. ... development ...
entrepreneur ...

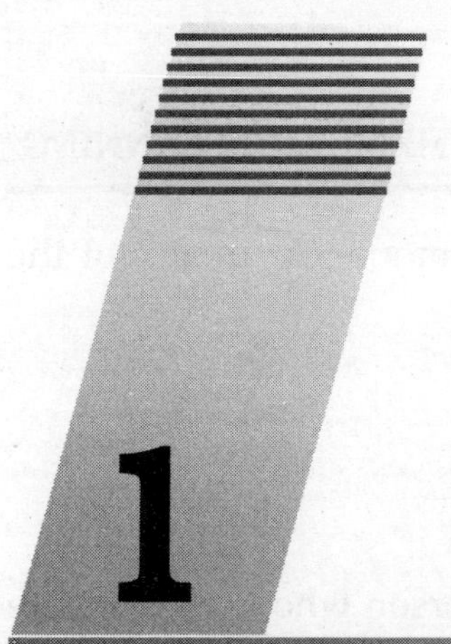

1 ENTREPRENEUR AND ENTREPRENEURSHIP

The word 'entrepreneur' has been taken from the French language, and it originally means an organiser of musical or other entertainments.

In the early 16th century, it was applied to those who were engaged in military expeditions. It was extended to cover civil engineering activities such as construction in the 17th century. It was only in the beginning of the 18th century that the word was used to refer to economic aspects. In this way, the evolution of the concept of entrepreneur is considered over more than four centuries old.

The term 'entrepreneur' is used in various ways and views. Broadly the three main views are:

1. Entrepreneur as a risk bearer

'Richard Cantillon' (Irish) was the first person who introduced the term 'entrepreneur' and his unique risk-bearing function in economics in the early 18th century. He defined entrepreneur as an agent who buys factors of production at certain prices in order to combine then into a product with a view to selling it at uncertain prices in future. Thus, it is a risk bearing activity.

2. Entrepreneur as an organiser

Jean-Baptiste say, developed the concept of entrepreneur by associating it with the functions of co-ordination, organization and supervision. According to him an entrepreneur is one who combines the land of one, the labour of another and capital of yet another and thus produces a product. By selling the product in the market, he pays interest on capital, rent on land and wages to labourers and what remains is his/her profit. Thus an entrepreneur is an organiser.

3. Entrepreneur as an innovator

''Joseph A. Schumpeter'' in 1934, assigned a crucial role of 'innovation' to the entrepreneur. He considered economic development as a dynamic change brought by entrepreneur by instituting new combinations of factors of production, i.e., innovations.

The introduction of new combination of according to him, may occur in any of the following forms:

(a) Introduction of new product in the market.

(b) Use of a new production technology.

(c) Opening of a new market.

(d) Discovery of a new source of supply of raw materials.

Definition. Thus an Entrepreneur can be defined as a person who tries to create something new, Organises production and undertakes riskes and handles economic uncertainity involved in enterprise, e.g., Ambani, Tata, Birla, Modi, Dalmia etc.

Characteristics of an Entrepreneur

1. Hard worker
2. Desire for high achievement
3. Independence
4. Foresight
5. Highly optimistic
6. Good organiser
7. Innovative
8. Urge to take calculated risk
9. Self-confidence
10. Seeing and acting on opportunities
11. Managerial skills
12. Good communication skills
13. Imaginative thinking
14. Emotional tolerance

Difference between Entrepreneur and a Manager

Points	Entrepreneur	Manager
1. Motive	The main motive of an entrepreneur is to start a venture by settingup an enterprise for his personal gratification	Main motive of a manager is to render his services in an enterprise already set up by some one else.
2. Status	Owner	Servant
3. Risk bearing	Assumes all risks and uncertainty involved in running the enterprise	Manager does not bear any risk involved in the enterprise.
4. Rewards	Profits (but highly uncertain and not fixed)	Salary (certain and fixed).
5. Innovation	Entrepreneur himself thinks over what and how to produce goods to meet the changing demands of the customers. Hence, he acts as an innovator/change agent.	A manager simply executes the plans prepared by the entrepreneur.
6. Qualification	An entrepreneur needs to possess qualities and qualifications like	A manager needs to possess distinct qualifications in

	high achievement motive, orginality in thinking, foresight risk bearing ability etc.	terms of sound knowledge in management theory and practice.

TYPES OF ENTREPRENEURS

Clarence Danhof classified entrepreneurs into four types on the basis of development stages – (At the initial stage of economic development, entrepreneur have less initiative and drives and as economic development proceeds, they become more innovating and enthusiastic).

1. Innovating entrepreneurs

He is one who introduces new goods, inaugurates new method of production, discovers new market and reorganises the enterprise. It is important to note that such entrepreneurs can work only when a certain level of development is already achieved and people look forward to change and improvement.

2. Initative entrepreneurs

There are characterised by readiness to adopt successful innovations inaugurated by innovating entrepreneurs. Imitative entrepreneurs donot innovate the changes themselves, they only imitate techniques and technology innovated by others. Such types of entrepreneurs are particularly suitable for the under-developed regions for bringing a mushroom drive of imitation of new combinations of factors of production already available in developed regions.

3. Fabian entrepreneurs

They are characterised by very great caution in experimenting any change in their enterprise. They imitate only when it becomes perfectly clear that failure to do so would result in a lose of the relative position in the eterprise.

4. Drone entrepreneurs

These are characterised by a refusal to adopt opportunities to make changes in production formula even at the cost of severely reduced returns relative to other like producers. Such entrepreneurs may ever suffer losses but they are not ready to make changes in their existing production methods.

OTHER TYPES

1. Solo operators

These are the entrepreneurs who essentially work alone and if needed at all, employ a few employees. In the beginning most of the entrepreneurs start their enterprises like them.

2. Active partners

These are the entrpreneurs who start or carry on their enterprise as a joint venture. Entrepreneurs who only contribute funds to one enterprise but do not actively participate in business activity are called simply 'partners'.

3. Inventors

Such entrepreneurs with their competence invent new product. Their basic interest lies in research and innovative activities.

4. Buyers

These are those entrepreneurs who do not like to bear much risk. Hence, in order to reduce risk involved in setting up a new enterprise, they like to buy the ongoing one.

5. Life timers

These entrepreneurs take business as an integral part to their life. Usually, the family enterprise and business.

INTRAPRENEUR

A new breed of entrepreneurs is coming to the fore in large industrial organizations. They are called, 'Intrapreneurs'. They emerge from within the confines of an existing enterprise. In big organization, the top executives are encouraged to catch hold of new ideas and then convert these into products through R and D activities within the framework of organization.

Table : *Difference between Entrepreneur and Intrapreneur*

	Entrepreneur	Intrapreneur
1. Dependency	An entrepreneur is independent in his operations	An intrapreneur is dependent on the entrapreneur i.e., the owner
2. Raising of funds	An entrepreneur himself raises funds required for the organi-zation	He doesn't raises fund for the organisation
3. Risk	Entrepreneur bears the risk involved in the business	An intrapreneur does not fully bear the risk involved in the organization
4. Operation	An entrepreneur operates from outside	An intrapreneur operates from within the organisation

ENTREPRENEURSHIP

DEFINITION

1. Entrepreneurship is the process of identifying opportunities in the market place, marshalling the resources required to pursue these opportunities and investing the resource for long term gains.
2. Entrepreneurship is the purposeful activity of an individual or a group of associated individuals undertaken to initiate, maintain and increase profit by production or distribution of economic goods and servicer. (Entrepreneurship is the set of activities performed by an entrepreneur) (e.g., management is what managers do).

Table : *Relation between Entrepreneur and Entrepreneurship*

Entrepreneur	Entrepreneurship
Person	Process
Organises	Organisation
Innovator	Innovation
Leader	Leadership
Risk bearer	Risk bearing
Visualises	Vision

Entrepreneurship is a process involving various actions undertaken to establish an enterprise.

CHARACTERISTICS/FEATURES OF ENTREPRENEURSHIP

1. Economic activity

Entrepreneurship is an economic function because it involves the creation and operation of an enterprise. It is basically concerned with production and distribution of goods and services.

2. Innovative function

Entrepreneurship is an innovative function as it involves doing things in a new and better way.

3. Goal oriented/purposeful activity

The entrepreneur who creates and operates an enterprise seeks to earn profits through satisfaction of needs of customers.

4. Risk bearing function

Risk is an inherent and inseparate element of entrepreneurship. He assumes the uncertanity of future and possibility of loss in pursuit of profits.

5. Organising function

An entrepreneur brings together various factors of production. He co-ordinates and controls the efforts of all the persons engaged in his enterprise. Therefore, he is an organisation builder.

6. Dynamic process

Entrepreneurs thrives on changes in the environment which bring useful opportunities for business. Flexibility is the hallmark of a successful entrepreneur.

ROLE OF ENTREPRENEURSHIP/ENTREPRENEURS IN ECONOMIC DEVELOPMENT OF INDIA

(Economic development essentially means a process of upward change where by the per capital income of a country increases over a long period of time.)

The economic history of the presently developed countries like America, Germany, Japan leads to support the fact that the economy is an effect for which entrepreneurship is the cause. The crucial role played by the entrepreneurs in the development of the western countries has made the people of under-developed countries too much conscious of the significance of entrpreneurship for economic development.

Now people have began to realise that for achieving the goal of economic development, it is necessary to increase entrepreneurship both qualitatively and quantitatively in the country. It is only active and enthusiastic entrepreneurs who fully explore the potentialities of the country's available resources land, tech., capital, material etc.

The role of entrepreneurship in economic development varies from economy to economy depending upon its material resources, industrial climate and the responsiveness of the political system to the entrepreneural function. The entrpreneurs contribute more in favourable opportunity conditions.

1. Thus in underdeveloped/developing regions, due to lack of funds and skilled labour, the atmosphere is less conducive for innovative entrepreneurs.
2. Under the conditions of paucity of funds and the problem of imperfect market, the entrepreneurs are bound to launch their enterprises on a small scale. Also initiator entrpreneurs are preferred in such regions. Thus, initation of innovations introduced in developed regions on a massive scale bring about rapid economic-developement in underdeveloped/developing regions.
3. Further India aims at decentralized industrial structure to reduce regional imbalances in levels of economic development.
4. Generation of employment
5. Balanced regional development
6. Improvement in standard of living
7. Backward and forward linkages

8. Creator of wealth (securities, issues etc.). Thus, small scale entrepreneurship in such industrial structure plays an important role to achieve balanced regional development, generation/creator of wealth etc.

Important role that entrepreneurship plays in the economic development of our economy (India) are:

1. Improvement in per capita income

Entrepreneurs locate and exploit opportunities. They convert the latent and idle resources like land, labour and capital into national income and wealth in the form of goods and services. They help increase Net National Product and Per Capita Income in the country.

2. Generation of employment

Entrepreneur generate employment both directly and indirectly. By starting their business they present an opportunity to others for work by offering jobs.

3. Balanced regional development

Entrepreneurs help to remove the regional disparities in the economic development of areas. They set up industries in backward areas to avail various substitutes and bring up the development of that region.

4. Improvement in living standards

Entrepreneur set up industry which introduce new products on a mass scale. There are at lower costs and this help to improve the standard of life of a common man.

5. Economic independence

Entrepreneurship is essential for national self reliance. Industrialists help to manufacture substitutes of imported products thereby reducing dependence on foreign countries. These businessmen also export products thereby earning foreign exchange for the country.

Entrepreneurship does not emerge and grow spontaneously. Their are various factors having both positive and negative influence on the growth of entrepreneurship. (Positive influence imply facilitating and conducive conditions wheras negative influences refer to factors inhibing the emergence of enterpreneurship).

Facilitating Factors	Barriers
1. Technical knowledge	1. Lack of technical skills
2. Entrepreneurial training	2. Lack of market knowledge
3. Market contacts	3. Lack of business knowledge
4. Family business	4. Time pressure and distractions
5. Availability of capital	5. Legal and bureaucratical contraints

6. Successful role models
7. Local manpower
8. Government and institutional support

6. Patent inhibitions
7. Political instability
8. Non-cooperate attitude of banks and other institutes

Factors Influencing Entrepreneurship

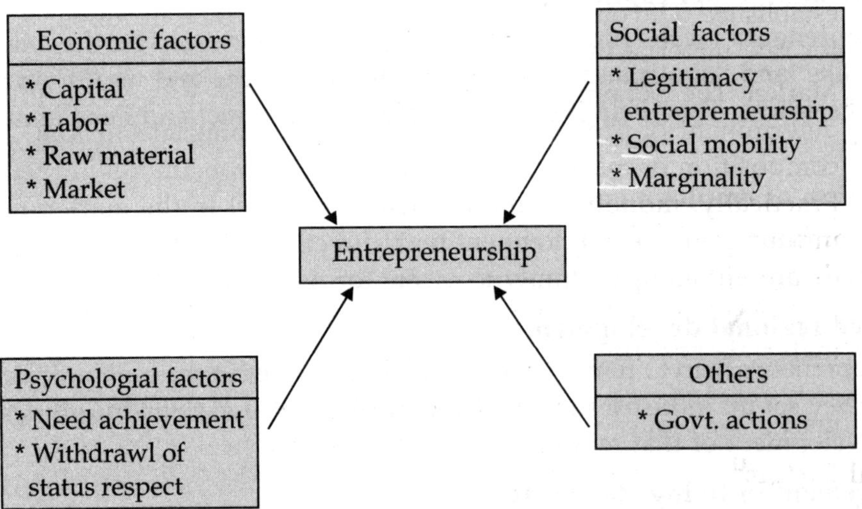

Fig. Factors influencing entrepreneurship

I. Economic conditions

Economic environment exercises the most direct and immediate influence on entrepreneurship. Capital labour, raw materials and markets are the main economic factors.

(a) **Capital.** It is one of the most important prerequisites to establish an enterprise. Availabity of capital facilitates the entrepreneur to bring together the land of one, machine of another and raw material of yet another to combine them to produce goods. With an increase in capital investment, capital-output ratio also increases. This results in increase in profit which ultimately goes to capital formation. This suggests that as capital supply increases, entrepreneurship also increases (e.g., Russia – how lack of capital for industrial pursuits impeded entrepreneurship).

(b) **Labour.** The quality rather than quantity of labour is another factor which influence the emergence of enterprise. Adam Smith considered division of labour as an important element in economic development. According to him, division of labour, which itself depends upon the sizes of the market leads to improvement in the productive capacities of labour due to an increase in the dexterity of labour. (But it appears that one labor problem clearly does not prevent entrepreneurship from emerging, for example, the problem of low cost immobile labour can be circumvented by plunging ahead with capital intensive technologies, as Germany did.)

(c) **Raw Materials.** The accessity of raw material for establishing any industrial activity, is indisputable. In the absence of raw materials, no enterprise can be established. Of course in some cases technological innovation can compensate for raw material inadequacy e.g., Japan.

(d) **Market.** The fact remains that the potential of the market constitutes the major determinant of probable rewards for entreprenurial function. The size and composition of market both influence entrepreneurship in their own ways. Practically, monopoly in a particular product in the market become more influential for entrepreneurship than a competitive market. However, the disadvantages of competitive market can be cancelled to some extent, by improvement in transportation system, facilitating the movement of raw materials and finished goods and increasing the demand for goods. For example, Germany and Japan are prime e.g., where rapid improvement in market was followed by rapid entrepreneurial activities.

II. Social Factors

Social environment in a country excercises a significant impact on the emergence of entrepreneurship. The various sub factor are:

(a) **Legitimacy of entrepreneurship.** The social factors give emphasis to the relevance of a system of norms and value, within a sociocultural setting for the emergence of entrepreneurship. This system is referred to as "legitimacy of entrepreneurship" in which the degree of approval or disapproval granted entrepreneural behaviour influences its emergence and characteristics if it does not emerge. Some scientists call it appropriate social climate for entrepreneurship and some call it cultural sanctions.

(b) **Social mobility.** It invloves the degree of mobility, both social and geographical and the nature of mobility channles within a system. Some are of the view that a high degree of mobility is conducive to entrepreneurship (e.g., openness of a system and need for flexibility in role relations imply the need for the possibility of mobility within a system for entrepreneurship development). In contrast, there is another group of scholars who express the view that a lack of mobility possibilities promotes entrepreneurship. The third opinion is a combination of first two, i.e., the need for both flexibility, the denial of social mobility. Thus a system should not be too rigid nor too flexible. (If too flexible individual will move towards other roles, if too rigid, entrepreneurship will be restricted alongwith other activities).

(c) **Marginality.** A group of scholars hold a strong view that social marginality also promotes entrepreneurship. They believe that individuals or groups on the perimeter of a given social system or between two social system provide the personnel to assume the entrepreneurial role. They may be drawn from religious, cultural, ethnic or migrant minority groups and their marginal, social position is generally believed to have psychological effects which make entrepreneurship particularly attractive for them.

III. Psychological Factors

(a) **Need achievement.** e.g., David Mc Clelland's theory of need achievement. According to him high need of achievement is the major influencing factor for entrepreneurship development therefore if the average level of need achievement in a socieity is relatively high, one would expect a relatively high amount of entrepreneurship in that society. Mc Clelland says that need achievement can be developed through the intensive training programmes.

(b) **Withdrawl of status respect.** Hagen attributed the withdrawal of status respect of a group to the genesis of entrepreneurship (e.g., Japan developed sooner than any non-western socierity except Russia due to two historical differences. First, Japan had been free from 'colonial disruption' and secondly, the repeated long continued withdrawal of expected status from important groups (like Samurai) in her society drove them to retraction which caused them to emerge alienated from traditional values with increased creativity. This very fact led them to the technological progress entrepreneurial roles). Hagen believes that the initial condition leading to eventual entrepreneurial behaviour is the loss of status by a group. He postulates that four types of events can produce status withdrawal.

(i) The group may be displaced by force
(ii) It may have, its valued symbols denigrated
(iii) It may drift into a situation of status inconsistency
(iv) Not accepted the expected status on migration in a new society

He furthes prostulates that withdrawl of status respect would give rise to four possible reactions and create four personality types :

(i) **Retreatist.** He who continues to work in a society, but remains different to his work and position.

(ii) **Ritualist.** He who adopts a kind of defensive behaviour and acts in the way accepted in his society but no hopes of improving his position.

(iii) **Reformist.** He is a person who forms a rebellion and attempts to establish a new society.

(iv) **Innovator.** He is a creative individual and is likely to be an entrepreneur.

Hagen maintains that once status withdrawl has occured, the sequence of change in personality formation is set in motion. He refers that status withdrawal takes a long period of time – as much as five or more generations to result in the emergence of entrepreneurship.

OTHERS

Govt. actions. The government by its actions or failure to act also does influence both the economic and non-economic factors for entrepreneurship. By creating basic facilities, utilities and services and by providing incentives and concessions, the government can provide the prospective entrepreneurs a facilitative socio-enonomic setting. Such conducive setting minimizes the risks which the entrepreneurs are to encountes.

Various factor stated above for emergence of entrepreneurship are interlocking, mutually dependent and mutually reinforcing. The various factors influencing the emergence of entrepreneurship can be put in a model developed by Abdul Aziz Mahmud (Model 1).

Integrated-contextual Model of Entrepreneurship

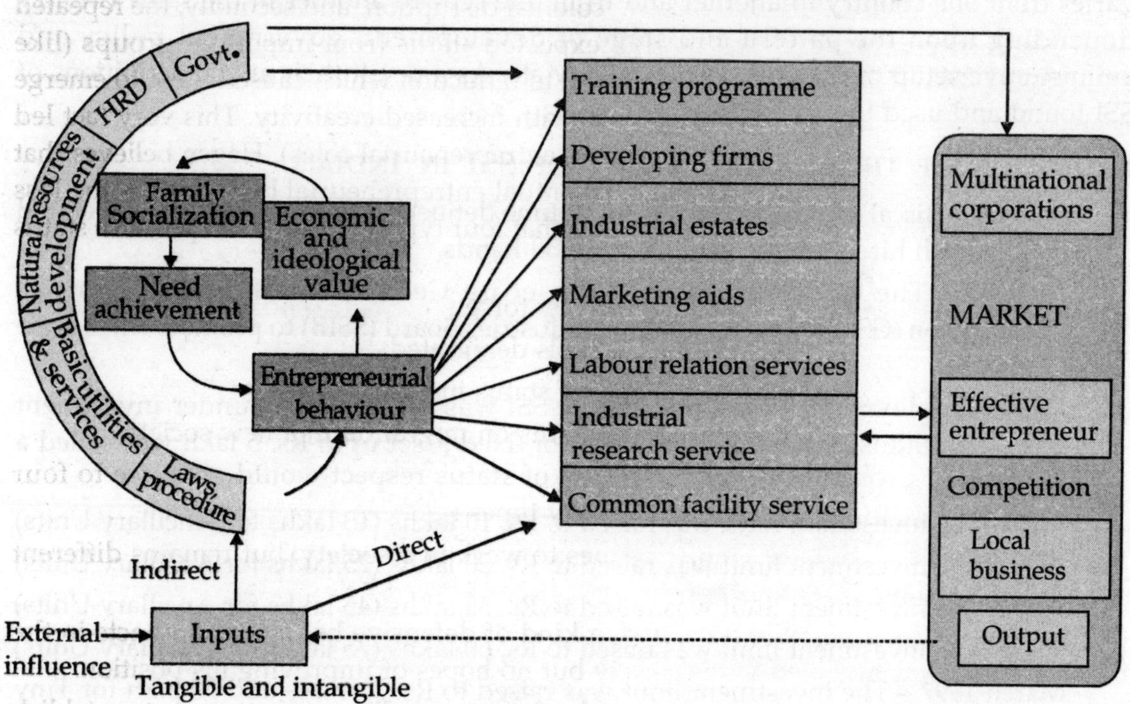

Model 1 : A model of factors influencing the emergence of entrpreneurship.

2 SMALL SCALE INDUSTRIES (SSI)

Small business enterprises exist in every country. But is a developing country like India the small scale sector occupies a special place in the industrial structure. In our country manpower is abundant but capital is relatively scarce. So SSI's tends to be labor intensive.

Small scale industry comprises of a variety of undertakings. The definition of SSI varies from one country to another and from one type to another in the same country depending upon the pattern and stage of development, government policy and aministrative setup of the particulars country etc. As a result their are 50 definitions of SSI found and used in 75 countries.

Evolution of the Legal Concept of SSI in India

1950 – The fiscal commission for the first time defined a SSI as one which is operated mainly with hired labour usually 10 to 50 hands.

1954-55 – The Government of India set up Central Small Scale Industries Organisation (CSSIO) and Small Scale Industries Board (SSIB) to promote small scale industries.

1960 – Employment criterion to define SSI was dropped and under investment criteria an industry having gross value of fixed asset upto Rs. 5 lakh was called a SSI.

1975 – The investment limit was raised to Rs. 10 lakhs (15 lakhs for Ancillary Units)

1980 – The investment limit was raised to Rs. 20 lakhs (25 lakhs for Ancillary Units)

1985 – The investment limit was raised to Rs. 35 lakhs (45 lakhs for Ancillary Units)

1995 – The investment limit was raised to Rs. 60 lakhs (75 lakhs for Ancillary Units)

March 1997 – The investment limit was raised to Rs. 3 crores and 50 lakh for Tiny Units

1999 – 2000 The investment limit was reduced to Rs. 1 crore.

2007 – Limit is 1 crore only

(An ancillary unit is one which sells not less than 50% of its manufactures to one or more industrial unit.)

CHARACTERISTICS OF SSI

1. A small scale unit is generally **one-man show.** Even the small units which run by a partnership firm or company, the activities are mainly carried out by one of the partners. The others are sleeping partners, who mainly assist in providing funds.
2. In case of SSI, the owner himself is a manager also. Thus these units are managed in a **personalized fashion.** The owner takes effective partcipation in all matters of business decision making.
3. The **scope of operation** of SSI is generally localised, catering to the local and regional demands.
4. **SSI are fairly, labour intensive** with comparatively smaller capital investments.
5. **Small units use indigenous resources and therefore can be located any-where, subject** to the availability of these resources like raw material, labout etc.
6. Using local resources, **small units are decentralized** and dispersed to rural areas. Thus, the developement of SSI in rural areas promotes more balanced regional development.
7. SS. units are **more change susceptible and highly reactive** and receptive to socio-economic conditions. They are more flexible to adopt changes like introduction of new products, new method of production new markets etc.

SCOPE

The scope of SSI is quite vast covering a wide range of activities requring less sophisticated technology. Important activities of SSI are–

- Manufacturing activities
- Servicing activities
- Retailing activities
- Financial activities
- Wholesale business
- Construction activities
- Infrastructural activities (e.g., transportation, communication etc.)

In orders to strengthen the scope for SI development in the country, the Govt. of India has, along with its other assistance programmes, annonced its reservation policy for small sector in the country. There are 824 items reserved for exclusive production in the small scale sector.

The number of SSI has grown from 2.96 lacks in 1977-78 to more than 30 lakhs in 2001-02.

OBJECTIVES

1. To generate immediate and large scale employment opportunities with relatively low investment.
2. To encourage dispersal of industries to all over country covering small towns, villages and economically lagging regions.
3. To promote balanced regional development in the whole country.
4. To improve the level of living of people in the country.
5. To encourage effective mobilization of country's untapped resources.

RELATIONSHIP BETWEEN SSI AND LARGE SCALE INDUSTRY (LSI)

The relationship between SSI and LSI can be seen in various respects. The complementary relationships are

1. Competitive

SSI can compete with large industry in certain circumstances and in selected products, e.g., bricks tiles, fresh baked goods and perishable edibles, preserved fruits, goods requiring small engineering. goods, items demanding craftsmanship and artisty.

2. Supplementary

SSI can fill in the gaps between large scale production and standard outputs caused by large scale units (e.g., SSI of tricycle factory along with cycle company).

3. Complementary

Many SSI produce intermediate products for large units. Under complementary relationship, small units function under the flagship of large units and enjoy the advantage of protected market for their products (e.g., seat covers, dust covers for electronic item).

4. Initiative

Attracted by the high profit of large units, small units can also take initiative to produce the particular product. If succeded, the small unit grows to large unit over a period of time.

5. Servicing

Small industries also provide servicing and repairing shops for the products of large units. For example, in areas like TV, radio, refrigerator, watches, cycles and motor vehicles.

6. Merchandising

Some small scale units disribute and sell there products through large scale units, for example, Hindustan Lever distributes soaps and cosmetics produced by some small firm. Footwear, electronics item, etc. manufatured by small units are marketed by large units.

7. Anciliarisation

Many large firms purchase components, parts and accessories from small firms which serve as ancillary units, for example, Maruti buys some components and accessories used in Maruti cars, from ancillary units.

Difference between SSI and LSI

SSI	LSI
Personal	Impersonal
Local area of operation	Wide area
Labor intensive	Capital intensive
Small fixed investment	Large investment
Decentralised location	Centralised location
Poprietorship and partnership	Joint stock company
Small uneconomic size	Large economic size
Unorganised labor	Organised labor

TYPES OF SSI

1. Manufacturing industries

Industries producing complete services for direct consumption and also processing units.

2. Feeder industries

Specialising in certain types of products and service, e.g., casting, electroplating, welding etc.

3. Servicing industries

Covering light repair shops necessary to maintain mechanical equipment.

4. Anciliary to large units

Producing parts and components and rendering services.

5. **Mining or quarrying**

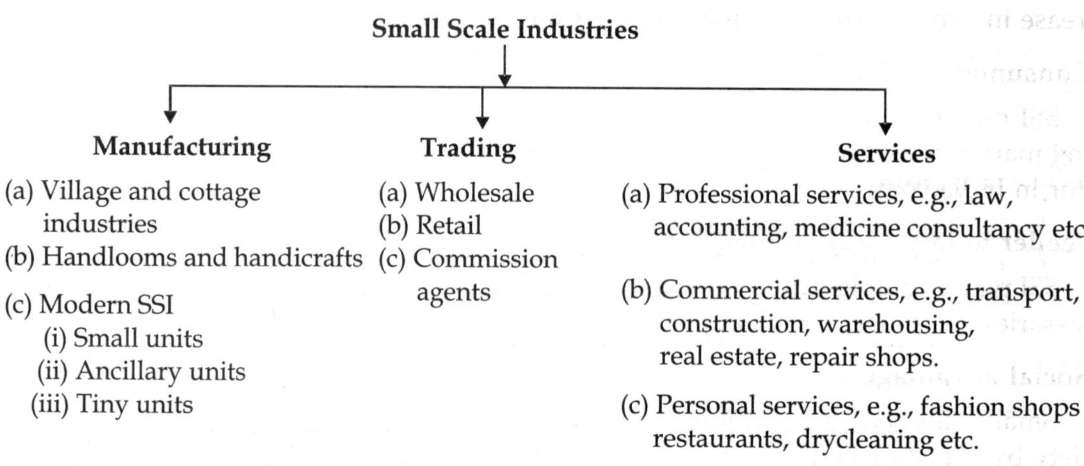

ROLE OF SSI IN INDIA ECONOMY

1. Employment

SSI use labor intensive techniques and therefore provide employment on a large scale, SSI accounts for 75% of the total employment in the industrial sector. SSI is provide self-employment to artisans, technically qualified persons and professionals. There industries also offer employment to farmer when they are idle.

2. Optimisation of capital

SSI requires less capital per unit of output and provide quick returns on investment due to shorter gestation period small scale units help to molatise small and scattered savings and channelise them into industrial activities.

3. Balanced regional development

SSI promote decentralised development of industries. They help to remove, regional disparities by industrialising rural and backward areas. They also help to improve the standard of living in suburban and rural areas.

4. Mobilization of local resources

SSI help to mobilise and untilise local resources like small savings, entrepreneurial talent etc. which might otherwise remain idle and unutilized. These industries facilitate the growth of local entrepreneurs and self-employed professional in small towns and villages.

5. Export promotion

SSI help in reducing pressure on the country's balance of payments in two ways. First they do not require imports of sophisticated machinery or raw materials. Secondly,

SSI can earn valuable foreign exchange through exports. There has been a substantial increase in exports from the small scale sector.

6. Consumer surplus

SSI now produce a wide range of mass conception items. Ones 5000 products are living manufactured in small scale sector. About one-half of the output of manufacturing sector in India comes from small scale industries.

7. Feeder to large scale industries

SSI play a complementary role to large scale sector. They provide parts, components, accessories etc. to large scale industries. They serve as ancillary units.

8. Social advantage

Small scale sector contributes towards the development of a socialistic pattern of society by reducing concentration of income and wealth. They provide as honourable and independent living to people with limited resources. They facilitate wide participation of public in the process of development.

9. Share in industrial production

SSI contribute more than one-half of the total industrial production in India. About 5000 products are manufactured in the small scale sector.

10. Development of entrepreneurship

Small scale units have helped to develop a class of entrepreneur. These units facilitate self-employment and spirit of self-reliance in the society.

PROBLEMS OF SSI

1. Problem of raw material
2. Problem of finance
3. Problem of marketing
4. Out dated technology
5. Poor project planning
6. Inadequate infrastructure
7. Others problems – shortage of trained staff, unorganised nature of operation etc.

1. Problem of raw material

There is scarcity of raw materials as well as poor quality and high costs. Since the emergence of modern small scale industries producing sophiticated items the problem of raw material has taken a major proportions. The small units that use imported raw material face this difficulty more on account of procurement of material or their costs.

2. Problem of finance

The problem of finance in SSI is mainly due to two reasons. Firstly, due to scarcity of capital and secondly, due to weak credit worthiness of small units in our country. Due to their weak economic base, SSI's find it difficult to take financial assistance from the commercial banks and financial institution etc.

3. Problem of marketing

The small units do not possess any elaborate marketing division. As a consequence there product does not get due favour compared to the products of large scale units.

4. Outdated technology

Most of the SSI depend upon old techniques and equipment. Due to limited capacity and capital, they find it very difficult to modernise their plant and increase thier quality of productions. Productivity also tends to be low.

5. Poor project plan

In the absence of education and experience small scale business often depend upon consultants. They do not fully understand project details. Due to poor planning of projects, cost and time overruns arise.

6. Inadequate infrastructure

Insufficient quality and quantity of transportation, communications and other basic services particularly in backward areas is another problems. Infrastructural gap results in underutilisation of capacity and occurence of wastages.

7. Other problems

In addition to the above stated problems in SSIs are constrained by numerous other problem like shortage of trained technicians, technological obsolescence, unorganised nature of operations etc.

ESTABLISHING A SMALL ENTERPRISE STEPS IN STARTING A BUSINESS VENTURE

Setting up of a new business enterprise is a very challenging and rewarding task. Several problems/decisions are involved in this task. Right from the selection of a right project/product upto the marketing of the product, numerous decisions have to be taken. The decision making process starts with project/product selection.

PROJECT

Meaning and definition. In simple words, "a project is an idea or plan that is intended to be carried out".

"A project is a scheme, design, a proposal of something intended or devised to be achieved".

"A project typically has a distinct mission that it is designed to achieve and a clear termination point, the achievement of the mission".

Thus a project can be defined as a scientifically evolved work plan devised to achieve a specific objective within a specified period of time.

While the projects can differ in their size, nature, objectives, time duration and complexity, yet they have three basic common attributes:

(a) A course of action,

(b) Specific objectives, and

(c) Definite time perspective.

(Every project has a starting point, and an end point with specific objective.)

FORMULATING PROJECT REPORT/BUSINESS PLAN

A project is a scheme, design or a proposal of something intended or devised. In simple term, project report or business plan is a written statement of what an entreprenur propose to take up.

It is like a kind of big road map to reach the destination determined by the entrepreneur.

TYPES OF PROJECTS

1. Quantifiable Projects

Projects whose benefits can be assessed in quantifiable term e.g., projects dealing with power generation etc.

Non-Quantifiable Project

Those project where quantifiable assessment of benefits is not possible, e.g., projects concerning with health, education etc.

2. 2nd basis–sectors; for example

1. Agriculture and Allied Sector
2. Irrigation and Power Sector
3. Industry and Mining Sector
4. Transport and Communication Sector
5. Social Service Sector
6. Miscellaneous Sector

3. 3rd basis–profit oriented and service oriented projects

Profit oriented

(i) New Projects
(ii) Development Project (Expansion)
(iii) Modernisation or Technology Projects
(iv) Diversification Projects

Service oriented projects

(i) Welfare Projects
(ii) Service Projects
(iii) R & D Projects
(iv) Educational Projects

IMPORTANCE OF A PROJECT REPORT

(i) Serves as a master plan: indicate goals.
(ii) Describes direction.
(iii) Forsees requirements.
(iv) Shows feasibility (from different angles).
(v) Indicates profitability (gives a indication of likely returns and benefits).
(vi) Helps in division making (important decisions can be taken with the help of a project report).
(vii) **Paves way for financial assistance**: It is on the basis of this report, that the financial institution make an appraisal and come to the conclusion.

(viii) **Ensures survival**: The survival of any business depends on the marketability of its products. The project report projects the demand and supply position, competitor position in the market, expected price etc., and thus ensures the survival of the business unit.

PRECAUTIONS IN PREPARING A PROJECT REPORT

(1) The prespective entrepreneur should always estimate his costs higher and his income lower than expected.

(2) He should not include any cost / price unless he himself has checked and verified that information. He must personally go into the market and confirm as much information as possible.

(3) If there is much time gap between the preparation of the project report and the implementaion of the project, then he should make necessary provision for cost education.

REASONS FOR THE FAILURE OF A PROJECT REPORT

(i) Failure to estimate the utilization capcity properly.

(ii) Not providing up-to-date information and supporting documents.

(iii) Not making adequate provisions for contingency.

(iv) Wrong selection of ownership form or not selecting as appropriate location.

ENCLOSURES IN PROJECT REPORT

(1) Certificate of educational qualification and experience.

(2) Copy of the plant layout with the map of factory, building and expected cost of building.

(3) Quotations for machinery and equipments.

(4) Copies of letters from prospective raw material suppliers.

(5) Copies of letters from future clients if any.

(6) Copy of the partership deed or any other relevant document.

(7) A schedule giving complete details of project implementation.

Main steps involved in the establishment of a small business venture are

I. Project Identification

It is the process of identifying opportunities for new business ventures. This process involves collection, compilation and analysis of relevant data for the ultimate purpose of choosing a suitable opportunity for investment. This process actually starts with idea generation.

In order to select the most promising project, the entrepreneur needs to generate a few ideas about the possible projects he can undertake. The project idea can be discovered from various sources : internal and external.

INTERNAL SOURCES

1. Knowledge of a person/experience.
2. Recombining the available elements in new and better ways.
3. Knowledge of potential customer needs.

EXTERNAL SOURCES

1. Success stories of others.
2. Project profiles for various industries.
3. Market surveys to know the trends.
4. Professional Journals, reports.
5. Visits to trade fairs, exhibitions etc.

Generation of business ideas or opportunities is also known as opportunity scanning and identification (OSI).

II. Project Selection

After generating ideas, it is necessary to evaluate them so as to identify the most appropriate idea/opportunity. This process is called 'Zeroing in process'. Following factors should be considered while selecting the product to be manufactured.

(i) Market potential.
(ii) Degree of competition.
(iii) An innovative idea which has greater project potential than an existing product.
(iv) Availability of raw material and technology.
(v) Resources and experience of the entrepreneurs in the line.
(vi) Govt. policies and regulation.
(vii) Suitability of the product to market requirements.

It is necessary to mention that each of these aspects has to be evaluated independently and in relation to each other. This forms a continuous and 'back and forth' process.

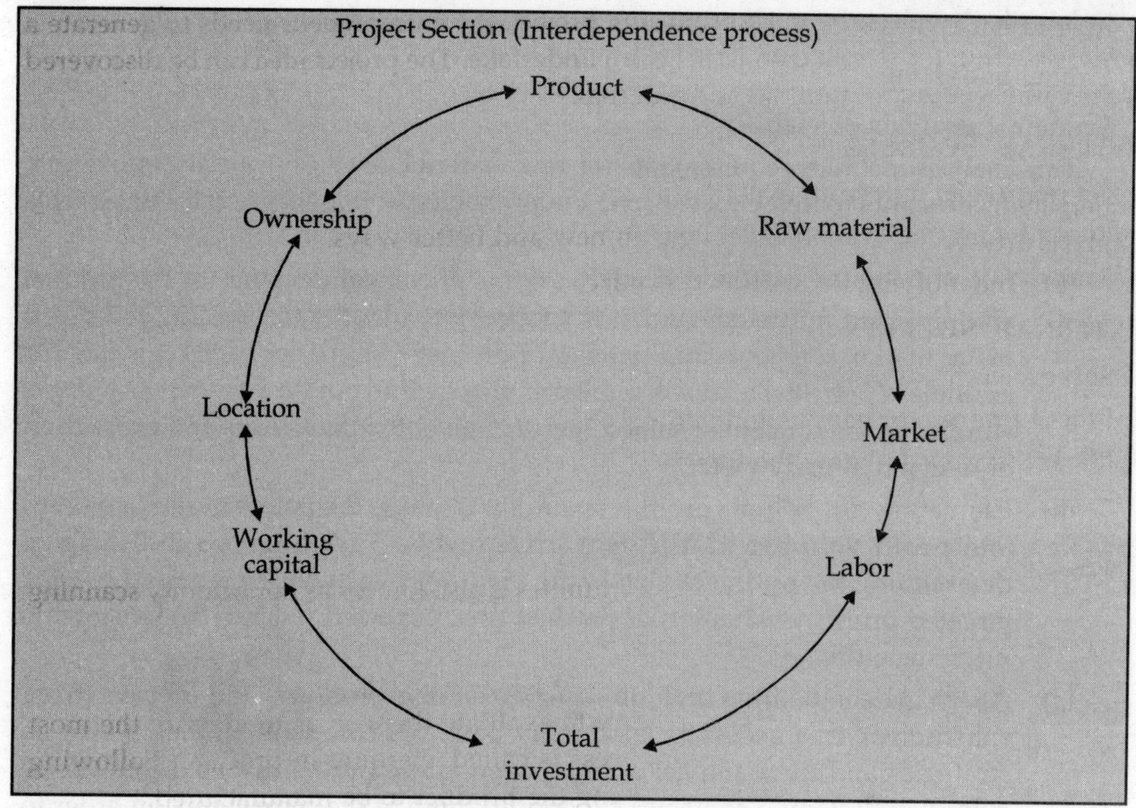

III. Project Appraisal (Project Evaluation)

In simple terms it means the assessment of project. It is done for both proposed and executed projects. In case of former, it is called, 'ex-ante analysis' and in case of latter 'post ante analysis'. (Here, project appraisal relates to a proposed project.)

Project appraisal is a costs and benefit analysis of different aspects of proposed project with an objective to adjudge its viability. An entrepreneur needs to appraise various alternative projects before allocating the scarce resources for the best project. (For appraising a project, its economic, financial, technical, market, material and social aspects are analysed.)

Appraisal of a project includes following analysis:

1. Economic analysis
2. Technical feasibility
3. Financial analysis
4. Managerial competence
5. Market analysis

6. Investment analysis

7. Capital budgeting.

1. Economic analysis or viability

This analysis includes requirements for raw material, level of capacity utilization, anticipated sales, anticipated expense and the probable profits. Steps/activities in this analysis are—

(a) Indentifying the market potential in terms of current demand for the product and projected future demand. it is necessary to identify the specific end users, major market segments and potential purchase volume for each segment. For example. a potential textbook publisher may be find out the number of students enrolled in the concerned subject, percentage of textbook users and proportion of demand already met.

(b) Estimating cost volume profit relationship to judge the potential sales volumes and profit volumes at different price levels. Such analysis will help in determining the optimum size of the venture, sales volume required to earn targeted profits, evaluation of product cost, expected revenue and a suitable price structure.

(c) Analysing competition both direct (from similar products) and indirect (from substitutes). It is necessary to identify potential competitors, their strength, strategies and there impact on the porposed venture. Such analysis will be helpful in designing strategies superior to those of the competitors. In order to judge the economic feasibility viability of a project considerable data is required. Such data includes:

 (i) Data relating to general economic trends such as per capita income, level of consumption, etc.

 (ii) Market data relating to demand pattern, competitors.

 (iii) Data related to price structure and discount pattern.

Market testings is important method of collecting market data.

Market testing. Interview, questionaires, now-a-days displaying the product at trade fairs, sample sales etc. are the modern methods.

2. Technical feasibility

It implies the availability of plant and machinery and technical know how to produce the product within the prescribed norms. It consists of:

(a) Identifying the technical specifications of the product in terms of its functional design, adaptability of new customer demand, durability, relability of performance, safety and standardisation.

(b) Finding out availability of necessary inputs, e.g., land, raw materials (both quantity and quality) plant machinery, technical skills, power and water, transport, communication facilities, service facilities, like repair shop etc. If technical know how is to be obtained from outside, arrangements made should be specified in the project report. Arrangements proposed for training of labor should also be mentioned. If the project requires any foreign collaboration, the terms and conditions thereof should be described.

(c) Preparing an outline of the manufacturing process including flow process charts.

(d) Testing the product through

  (i) Engineering studies relating to machines, tools and work-flow.

  (ii) Product development through blueprint, model, prototype.

  (iii) Product testing through laboratory and field study.

3. Financial analyis/financial feasibility

It comprises of the following aspects:

(a) **Assessment of total financial requirements (fixed and working capital).** Project costs consists of non-recurring (fixed) and recurring expenses (working). Fixed includes land and buildings, plant and machinery, furniture etc. The amount of fixed capital will depend on the scale of operations, type of technology, time of investment etc. Working capital or recurring expenses include raw materials, stock of finished goods, wages and salaries etc. It will depend upon the level of activity, terms of purchase and sale etc.

(b) **Determining source and costs of funds.** Once the total funds required are estimated appropriate source, need to be choosen to raise the required investment.

(c) **Analysing cash flow.** After estimating the amount of funds required, the anticipated flow of cash from the project are determined. For this purpose a cash flow statement is prepared.

(d) **Anticipating return on investment.** No project is financially feasible unless it generates a satisfactory yield on investment. Average earnings expected from the project over a specific period of time when divided by investment shows the return. Such return when compared with potential return from alternative, investment opportunities will help in deciding the acceptability or otherwise of the project.

4. Managerial competence

A proper assessment of the number and skills of staff required for the project is necessary. For this purpose an appropriate organisation structure is decided. Then the skills and talents required for staff w.r.t. structure are determined.

5. Market analysis

Before the production actually starts, the entrepreneur needs to anticipate the possible market for the product. He has to anticipate who will be the potential buyer for his product and where and when his product will be sold. (Production has no value for the producer unless it is sold.) There are various methods to anticipate potential market (konwn as demand forecasting). There are

(A) **Opinion polling method.** In this method, the opinions of the ultimate user i.e., consumers of the product is estimated

  (i) **Complete enumeration survey**. In this survey, the probable custmers of the product are approached and this probable demand for the product are estimated and then summed.

  (ii) **Sample survey**. Under this method, only some number of consumers out of their total population is approached and data on their probable demands for the product during the forecasted period are collected and summed.

  (iii) **Vicarious method**. Under this method, the consumers of the product are not approached directly but indirectly through some dealers who have a feel of their customers.

(B) **Life cycle segmentaion analysis.** In practice, a product sells slowly in the begining. Backed by sales promotion strategies over period, its sales pick up. In the due course of time, the peak sale is reached. After that point, the sales begins to decline. After some time, the product loses its demand and dies. This is natural death of a product. Thus, every product passes through its 'life cycle'. This is precisely the reason why firms go for new products one after another to keep the firm alive. Based on above, the product life cycle has been divided into the following five stages.

Introduction – Growth – Maturity – Salturation – Decline

The sales of the product varies from stage to stage and follows S-shaped curve as shown below.

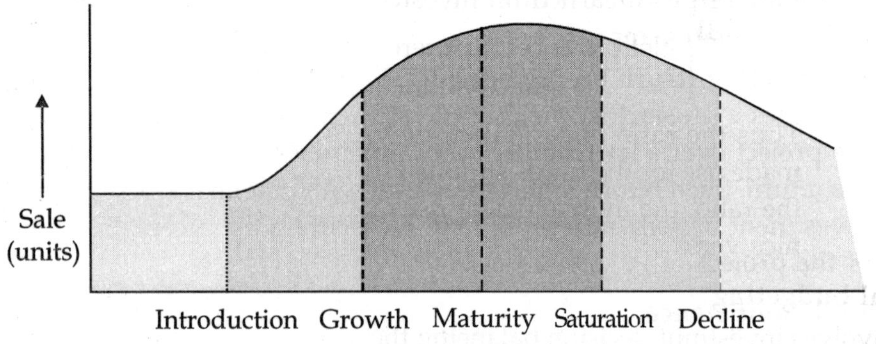

Fig. Product life cycle

Considering the above stages of a product life cylce, the sales at different stages can be aticipated.

6. Investment/Risk Analysis

Production of a new product or diversification both involve investment. The basic objective of every investment is to maximize profit. Thus, capital should be invested in those opportunities which show more prospects of profit. Proper investment analysis enables the entrepreneur to choose an investment out of a given set of alternatives.

Investment analysis primarily deals with the interpretation of the data incorporated in the profoma financial statements of a project and the presentation of data in a form in which it can be utilized for a comparative apprasisal of the projects. The technique of ratio analysis and capital budgeting have been used as the most important tools of investment analysis.

(a) **Ratio analysis**. A ratio shows the arithmetical relationship between two relevant figure, with the help of ratios we can reach useful conclusions about the profitability of investments made in the enterprise. Profitability rates are calculated by relating profits either to sales or to investments. They are usually expressed in percentages. profit is volume and profitability is a ratio. Following are some important profitability ratios in relation to investment decisions.

(i) **Return on proprietor's fund or net worth**. This ratio expresses the ratio of net profit after tax and interest to propritor's funds or net worth. Calculated as:

$$\left(\frac{\text{Net Profit after tax and interest}}{\text{Propriector's funds or net worth}}\right)$$

(ii) **Return on capital employed**. This ratio indicates the earning power of the capital employed in the business and point out to the owner the progress or deterioration in the earning capacity of the business. (It shows ratio of profit earned on invested capital). It is calculated as:

$$\left(\frac{\text{Net profit before interest and tax}}{\text{Capital employed}}\right) \times 100$$

Thus the ratio of capital employed indicates how the management has made use for the funds supplied by owner and creditors, Obviously higher the ratio, the more efficient use of the funds the enterprise is making and nice versa.

7. Capital budgeting

It involves investmnt decision balancing the sources and uses of funds for acquiring fixed capital assets like machines and equipments. The scarce capital is to be invested in the most profitable project. Various techniques of capital budgeting are:

(i) **Payback or payout period**. This tech. answers an investor's searching question as to how long he has to wait before the invested capital is recovered. The cash flow starts coming and accumulating. After a certain period of time the accumulated cash inflows become equal to the original investment made. At that point of time the payback occurs and the time it has taken for recovery is called Payback or Payout Period.

This method involves chosing that project which repays the initial investiment in the shortest period of time.

(ii) **Break-even analysis**. It is the analysis of finding out the production point, where income exactly equals expenses.

(iii) **How to find break-even**. Expenses to be incurred refer to cost. Cost is of two types: fixed and variable.

(a) **Fixed costs**. Are those that do not change with increase or decrease is production. No matter what the production is the fixed cost remain the same e.g. monthly rent paid for one factory, interest on long term loan etc. Even if there is zero production, the fixed cost will remain unchanged.

Though absolute fixed cost will remain unchanges but per unit fixed cost will vary with change in production. For example–

Month	**Total fixed cost**	**Production in units**	**Fixed cost per unit**
March	10,000 rent	400	10,000 ÷ 400 = 25 Rs.
April	10,000	500	10,000 ÷ 500 = 20 Rs.
May	10,000	200	10,000 ÷ 200 = 50 Rs.

So, fixed cost per unit decrease with increase in production and increase with decrease in production.

(b) **Variable costs**. These are expenses that change with volume of production. It varies proportionately with changes in production. Thus if production is zero, variable cost would be zero. The absolute total variable cost increases or decreases along with increase or decrease in production. But the variable cost per unit is constant at any level of production. For example-

Month	**Production (Units)**	**Total variable cost (cost of raw material)**	**Variable cost/Units**
March	1,000	50,000	50,000 ÷ 1,000 = 50
April	1,600	80,000	80,000 ÷ 1,600 = 50
May	1,500	75,000	75, 000 ÷ 1,500 = 50

There are some variable costs that do not vary proportionately with the change in production. In fact, there vary in varying degrees. As a result such costs are called semivariable, e.g., cost of telephone, electricity, etc. are billed on usage basis. In such cases, that proportion of expenses which continue even if production falls are called as fixed and expenses which increase or decrease as production increase or decrease are called variable costs.

After knowing sales and total cost in terms of fixed cost, now and variable cost the breakeven point can be calculated.

According to the simplest method, profit is the excess of sales over cost, i.e., sales – cost = profit. The calculation of break even point involves four steps. These are:

1. Segregation of fixed and variable costs.
2. Percentage of variable costs to sales.
3. Calculate the contribution or margin i.e., the difference between 100 and the percentage of variable cost to sales as worked out above.
4. Divide the fixed cost by the percentage of contribution or margin as worked out above. The calculated figure will be break-even point.

To calculate Break Even Point

For example, total sales of a enterprise is Rs. 8,00,000. The various costs are:

Items	Variable costs (Rs.)	Fixed costs (Rs.)
Raw material	80,000	—
Power	30,000	60,000
Wages	80,000	65,000
Administrative expenses	30,000	50,000
Selling expenses	40,000	10,000
Manufacturing expenses	20,000	25,000
Miscellaneous expenses	50,000	—
Total	3,20,000	2,10,000

Following the aforesaid four steps, we find:

1. Variable cost Rs. 3,20,000, fixed cost Rs. 2,10,000
2. Percentage of variable cost to sales = 3,20,000, 8,000,000 × 100 = 40%
3. Contribution or Margin = 100 – 40 = 60%
4. Break even point in terms of sales will be $\frac{2,10,000 \times 100}{60}$ = Rs. 3,50,000

So at a sale of Rs. 3,50,000 the enterprise will gain neither profit nor loss.

Break even chart

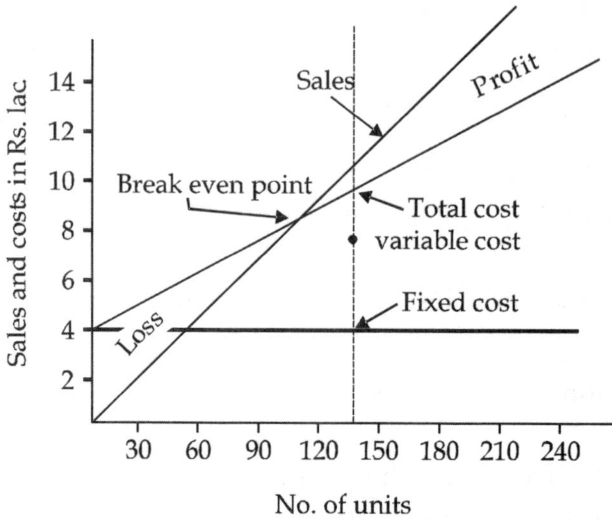

IV. **Project Formulation**

Project formulation is the systematic development of a project idea for the eventual purpose of arriving at an investment decision. It involves step by step investigation and development of project idea. This process involves the joint efforts of a team of experts. Each member of the project team should be fully familar with one broad strategy, objectives and other ingredients of the project.

A well formulated project is the best passport for obtaining the required assistance from financial institutions. Project formation will also be of great help in obtaining necessary clearance from the government.

Small entrepreneurs also need to draw the business plans because right from the conception of a business idea upto production involves numerous decisions to be taken.

Formulation of project report/business plan is one of the first stone to be laid down in setting up an enterprise.

"Project report or business plan is a written statement of what an entrepreneur proposes to take up. So it is an operating document".

The preparation of a project report is of great significance for an entrepreneur. First and foremost, the project report is like a road map. It describes the direction the enterprise is going in, what its goals are, where it wants to be and how it is going to get there. It also enables on entrepreneur to know that he is proceeding in the right direction. Banks and other financial institutions judge a project on the basics of feasibility report. The entrepreneur who asks for financial asistance has to submit such a report.

Project formulation devides the process of project development into eight distinct and sequential parts. There are

1. General information
2. Project description
3. Market potential
4. Capital costs and sources of finance
5. Assessment of working capital requirements
6. Other financial aspects
7. Economic and social variables
8. Project implementation

1. General information

This includes

(a) *Biodata of promoter*. Name, address, qualification, experience etc.

(b) *Industry profile*. Reference of industry to which project belongs, past performance, present status, problems etc.

(c) *Constitution and organisation*. Organization structure of the firm, its regitration under concerned authority.

(d) *Product deatails*. Product utility, product range, design, advertisment of product over its substitutes if any.

2. Project description

It covers

(a) *Site*. Location of enterprise, NOC from muncipal authority if in redidential area.

(b) *Physical infrastructure*. Availability of following items should be mentioned in report:

(i) *Raw material*. Requirement and sources.

(ii) *Skilled labour*. availability, arrangements for training.

(c) Utilities. These include

(i) *Power*. Requirement, land sanctioned.

(ii) *Fuel*. Requirement of coal, oil/gas and availability.

(iii) *Water*. Sources and quality of water.

(d) *Pollution control*. Scope of dump, sewage system and sewage treatment plant in case of industry producing emissions.

(e) *Communication system*. Availability of communication facilities, e.g., phone, fax etc.

(f) *Transport facilities*. Requirement for transport, mode, distance covered etc.

(g) Other common facilities. e.g., machine shops, welding shops, electrical repairs shops etc.

(h) *Production process.* Automatic, manual, mechanical, etc.

(i) *Machinery and equipment.* Complete list of item of machinery and equipments, indicating their size, type, cost and sources of supply.

(j) *Capacity of the plant.* Installed licensed capacity along with shift.

(k) *R and D.* Proposed R and D activities to be undertaken in future.

3. Market potential

The following aspects should be included

(i) *Demand and supply position.* State the total expected demand for the product and present supply position. Also mentioned should be how much gap will be filled by the proposed unit.

(ii) *Expected price.* Expected price of the product.

(iii) *Market strategy.* Arrangements made for selling the product.

(iv) *After sales service.* Depending upon the nature of the poduct provision made for after sales service should be stated.

4. Capital costs and sources of finance

An estimate of the various components of capital items like land and buildings, plant and machinery, installation costs, preliminary expenses, and margin for working capital should be given in the report.

5. Assessment of working capital requirements

The requirement for working capital and its sources of supply should be carefully and clearly mentioned in the project report.

6. Other financial aspects

In order to adjudge the profitability of the project to be set up, a projected profit and loss account indicating likely sales revenue, cost of production, allied cost and profit should be prepared. In addition break even analysis should also be included.

7. Economic and social variables

In view of the social responsibility of business, the abatement costs, i.e., the costs for controlling the environmental damage should be stated in the project. Besides the socio-economic benefits expected from the project should also be stated (e.g., employment generation, exports, ancillarisation, local resource utilization, development of the area etc.)

8. Project implementation

Every entrepreneur should draw an implementation scheme or a time-table for his project to ensure the timely completion of all activities involved in setting up an enterprise.

COMMON ERRORS IN PROJECT FORMULATION

Entrepreneurs often make errors while formulating project reports and business plans. Following are some of the important errors in project formulation.

1. Product selection

Some entrepreneurs commit mistakes by selecting a wrong product for their enterprise. They select the product without giving due attention to product related other aspects such as size of the product, market, competition, life cycle, availability of labor, raw material and technology, future demand etc.

2. Capacity utilization estimates

The entrepreneurs usually make over-optimistic estimates of capacity utilization. Their estimate are based on a completely false premises, with complete disregard to present enterprise performance, prevailing market condition, competition etc.

3. Technology selection

The requirement of technology (manual, machine or automatic) differs from product to product. Swayed by the imagined profit margin the entrepreneurs sometimes plan for a technology which is not possible to set up within the available finance. Thus failure is seen.

4. Selection of ownership form

Many business fail primarily because the ownership selected for the enterprise is not suitable.

5. Market study

Product is eventually made for sale in the market. Based on scanty information about the demand and supply of that product the entrepreneurs believe that their product has good market for selling. Their data is not accurate and based on human preference which change with time.

PROJECT SCHEDULING

This aspect also called as Network Analysis.

A network is a set of symbols connected with each other with a sequential relationship with each step making the completion of a project/event. A business plan or project involves various activities to be undertaken to convert it into an enterprise delays in the timely completion of activities may cause time, energy and money loss among other things. Hence, there is a need for dividing the sequential order of all activities of the project so as to accomplish the project economically in the minimum available time and with the limited resources. A numbers of network techniques have been developed for project scheduling. some of them are:

1. **PERT** – Programme Evaluation and Review Technique
2. **CPM** – Critical Path Method

3. **GERT** – Graphical Evaluation and Review Technique
4. **WASP** – Workshop Analysis Scheduling Programme
5. **LOB** – Line of Balance

Some of the above techniques are discussed in detail:

1. Programme Evaluation and Review Technique (PERT)

PERT was first developed as a Aid for completing Polaris Ballistic Missle Project in USA in Oct. 1958. It worked well in expediting the completion of the project from 7 years to 5 years. Since then, PERT has become very popular technique for project planning and control. In summary, it schedules the sequence of actitivies to be completed in order to accomplish the project within a short period of time. It helps reduce both the time and cost of the project.

Steps in PERT

(a) The activities involved in the project are drawn up in a sequential relationship to show what activity follows what.

(b) The time required for completing each activity of the project is estimated and noted on network.

(c) The critical activities of the project are determined.

(d) The variability of the project duration and probability of the project completion in a given time period are calculated.

Advantage of PERT

(a) It determines the expected time required for completing each activity.

(b) It helps complete the project within a given period of time.

(c) It helps management handle uncertainities involved in the project and thus, reduce the risk element in the project.

(d) It enables management to make optimum allocation of limited resources.

(e) It presses for the right action, at the right point and at the right time in the organization.

Limitation of PERT

(a) PERT network is mainly based on time estimate required for each activity. On account of wrong time estimated, the network is bound to become highly unrealistic.

(b) This technique also does not consider the resources required at different stages of the project.

(c) For effective control of a project by using PERT techniques requires frequent updating and revising the PERT calculation. But this provs quite a costly affair for the organisation.

2. **Critical Path Method (CPM)**

CPM was first developed in USA by the E.I Dupant Nemours & Co. in 1956 for doing periodic overhauling and maintenance of a chemical plant. It resulted in reducing the shut-down period from 130 hrs to 90 hrs and saved the company 1 million dollars. The CPM differentiates between planning and scheduling of the project. While planning referes to determination of activities to be accomplished, scheduling refers to introduction of time schedule for each acting of the project. The duration of different activities in CPM are deterministic. There is a precise known time that each activity in the project will take.

Advantages of CPM. Main advantages are:

(a) It helps in accelerating the time schedule of activities having sequential relationship.

(b) It makes control easier for the management.

(c) It identificer most critical elements in the project. Thus, the management is kept alert and prepared to pay due attention to the critical activities on the project.

(d) It makes better and detailed work schedule.

Limitations of CPM. Main disadvantages are:

(a) CPM operates on the assumption that there is a precise known time that each activity in the project will take. But, it may not be true in real practice.

(b) CPM time estimates may not be based on statistical analysis.

(c) CPM cannot be used as a dynamic controlling device for the simple reason that any change introduced will change the entire structure of network.

Table : *Difference between PERT and CPM*

PERT	CPM
1. Its origin is military	1. Its origin is industry
2. It is a probalistic model	2. It is a determinitic model
3. It average time	3. It does not average time
4. It is an event oriented approach	4. It is an activity oriented approach
5. It allows uncertainity	5. It does not allow uncertainity
6. It does not demarcate between critical and non critical activities	6. It demarcates between critical critical and non critical activities
7. It is suitable when reasonable precision is required	7. It is suitable when high precision is required

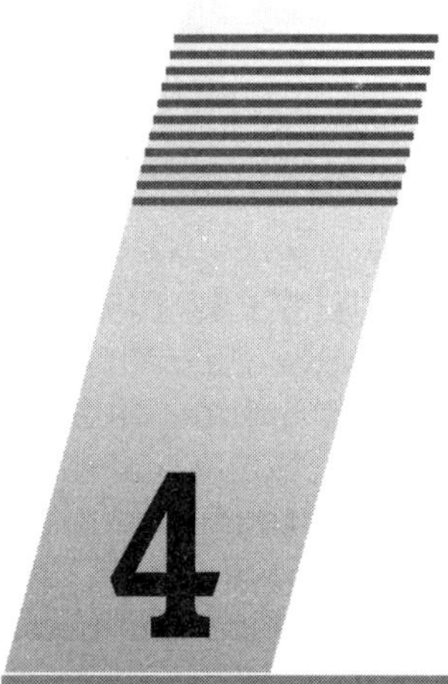

4 FORMS OF OWNERSHIP

An important decision which an entrepreneur has to take is the legal structure of his enterprise. This decision is important because the choice of ownership form affects the rights, duties and obligation of owners as well as tax liability.

THE MAIN FORMS OF OWNERSHIP ARE

1. **Sole proprietorship** *or individual entrepreneurship*

Is a business concern owned and operated by one person. He alone contributes the capital and skills and is solely responsible for the results of the enterprise.

ADVANTAGE

(i) **Simplicity** – Very easy to establish and dissolve a sole proprietorship, e.g., a shop owner.

(ii) Quick decisions.

(iii) **High secrecy** – His business secrets are known to him only.

(iv) Personal Touch.

(v) **Flexibility** – Complete freedom of action.

DISADVANTAGES

(i) Limited funds.

(ii) Limited skills.

(iii) Uncertain life.

2. Partnership firm

As a business enterprise expands beyond the capacity of a single person, a group of persons have to join hands together and supply the necessary capital and skills. Need to arrange more capital, provide better skills and avail of specialization led to the growth of partnership form of organization.

Definition. According to Sec. 4 of the Partnership Act 1932, partnership is "relation between persons who have agreed to share the profits of a business carried on by all or anyone of them acting for all".

CHARACTERISTICS

(i) Association of 2 or more persons, max. 10 in banking business and 20 for non-banking business.

(ii) **Contractural agreement**. Written or oral among the partners.

(iii) Sharing of profit and loss.

(iv) **Existence of lawful business**. Partnership is formed to carry on some lawful business and share its profits and loss. If the purpose it to carry some charitable works, it is not regarded as partnership.

(v) **Unlimited liability**. i.e., if the assets of the partership firm fall short to meet the firm's obligations, the partner's private assets will also be used for the purpose.

ADVANTAGES

(i) **Easily formed.** No cumbersome legal formalities.

(ii) Large financial resources (as more than one person).

(iii) Specialization and balanced approach.

(iv) **Flexibility of operations**. Not as versatile as propreitorship, a partership firm enjoys sufficient flexibility in its day-to-day operation. Partership is free from statutory control by the Govt. except the general law of the land. (change the function, operation product, add or delete partners etc. is possible).

(v) **Capacity for survival**. The firm can continue even after the death or insolvency of a partner if the remaining partners so desire. Risk of loss is diffused among two or more persons. Due to number of representatives (partners).

(vi) **Better human and public relations**. Personal touch maintained with employees, customers, Govt. etc.

DISADVANTAGES

(i) Limited resources.

(ii) Lack of harmony.

(iii) Public distrust.

(vi) **Unlimited ability**. Every partner is jointly and severally liable for the entire debts of the firm. He has to suffer not only for his own mistakes but also for the lapses and dishonesty of other partners. Private property of partners is not safe against the risk or business.

(v) **Non-transferability of shares.** No partner can transfer his share in the firm to an outsides without the unanimous consent of all the partners. This makes investment in a partership firm non-liquid and fixed. An individual's capital is blocked.

3. Joint Stock Company

A joint stock company is an incorporated and voluntary association of individuals with a distinctive name, perpetual succession, limited liability and common seal, and usually having a joint capital divided into transferable shares of a fixed value.

CHARACTERISTICS

(a) **Separate legal entity**. A company has an existence entirely distict from and independent of its members. It can own property and enter into contracts in its own name. It can use and be sued in its own name. The assets and liabilities of the company are not the assets and liabilities of the individual members and vice versa.

(b) **Artificial legal person.** A compnay is an artificial person created by law and existing only in contenplation of law. It is intangible and invisible having no body or soul. It is an artificial person because it does not come into existence through natural birth and it does not possess the physical attributes of a natural person. But like a natural person, it has rights and obligations in terms of law.

(c) **Perpetual succession**. A company enjoys continous or uninterupted existence and its life is not affected by the death or insolvency etc. of its members or directors. Being a creature of law a company can be dissolved only through the legal process of winding up.

(d) **Limited liability**. Liability of the members of a limited company is limited to the value of the shares subscribed to or to the amount of guarantee given by them (unlimited companies are an exception rather than the general rule). In a limited company members cannot be asked to pay anything more than what is due or unpaid on the shares held by them even if the assets of the company are insufficient to satisfy in full the claim of its creditors.

(e) **Transferability of shares**. The shares of a public limited company are freely transferable. They can be purchased and sold through the stock exchange. Every member is free to transfer his shares to anyone without the coursent of other members.

ADVANTAGES:

(i) **Limited liability.** The liability of shareholders, unless and otherwise stated, is limited to the face value of shares held by them or guarantee given by them.

(ii) **Perpetual existence**. Death, insanity or insolvency of shareholders or directors do not affect the compnay's existence. Company has separate legal entity with perpectual succession.

(iii) **Professional management**. In company business, the management is in the hands of the directors who are elected by the shareholders and are well experienced persons. In order to manage the day-to-day activities, salaried professional manager are appointed.

(iv) **Transferability of shares**. If the shareholders of a company are displeased with the progress of the business, they can sell their shares anytime. During all this change of ownership, the business continues to operate.

(v) **Diffusion of risk.** As the membership is very large, the whole business risk is divided among the several members of the company.

DISADVANTAGES

(i) **Lack of secrecy.** As per the legal provisions, a company has to make various statements available to the registrar of companies, financial institution, thus the secrecy of business comes down. It is further reduced when the company provides its annual report to the shareholders as the competitors do also find out the details of all financial data.

(ii) **Legal restrictions**. Compared to proprietorship and partnership, a company has to comply with more legal requirements.

(iii) **Management mischiefs**. Sometimes the managers and directors misuse the company resources for their personal benefits.

(iv) **Lack of personal interest**. Unlike proprietorship and partnership the day-to-day affairs of a company are looked after by salaried managers. Since they are the employees and not the owners, they hardly have personal interest and commitment in the company this may cause losses.

Mainly two types : Private Company and Public Company

Basis of difference	Private Company	Public Company
1. Members	Min. - 2, Max. - 50	Min. - 07, Max. - no limit
2. Directors	Min - 2	Min. - 03
3. Allotment of shares	It may commence allotment of shares before min. subscription has been applied for restricted by article	It cannot commence allotment of shares unless min. subscription has been applied for.
4. Transfer of shares		Shares freely trasferable
5. Filling of balance sheet	It need not file its balance sheet with the registrar	It must file its balance sheet with the registrar

6. Name	Pvt. Ltd.	Ltd.
7. Term of	Till retirement or resignation servive of director	1/3 of the members change every 2 years.

4. Co-operatives

This type of organisation is based on the philosophy of self help and mutual help. The basic line of difference is that a co-operative organisation aims at rendering in place of earning profits.

Definition. According to International Labour organisation co-operative organisation is an association of persons, usually of limited means, who have voluntarly joined together to achieve a common economics and through the formation of a democratically controlled business organisation making equitable distribution to capital required and accepting a fair share of risks and benefits of the undertaking.

It should have minimum of 10 members are no limit for maximum number. The members are the owners. They contribute capital to the organisation and get dividents. The liability of the owners is limited.

MAIN FEATURES

(a) **Voluntary organisation.** Co-operative organisation is voluntary association of person desirous of pursuing a common objective. They can come and leave the organisation at their own will without coercion or intimidation.

(b) **Service motive.** The primary objective of a co-operative society is to render services rather than to earn profits.

(c) **Capital and return thereon.** The capital is produced from its members in the form of share capital. A member can subscribe to max. of 10% of the subscribe total share capital or Rs. 1,000 whichever is higher. Shares cannot be transferred but surrendered to the organisation. The rate of dividends paid to the members/shareholders is restricted to 9% as per the Co-operative Societies Act, 1912.

(d) **Government control.** In India, the activities of co-operative societies are regulated by the Co-operative Societies Act, 1912 and the State Co-operative Societies Act 1912. Co-operative societies are required to submit their annual report and accounts to the Registrar of Co-operatives.

(e) **Democratic management.** The management of co-operative organisation is vested in the hands of the managing commitee elected by the members on the basis of 'one members one vote' irrespective of the number of shares held by any member. The general body of the members lays down the broad framework within the managing commitee has to function.

ADVANTAGES

(i) **Easy formation.** Any 10 adult persons can voluntarily form themselves into an association and get it registered with the registrar of co-operatives. Thus no ling and complicated legal formalities.

(ii) **Limited liability.** The liability of members is limited to the extent of their capital in the co-operative societies.

(iii) **Perpetual existence**. A co-operative society has a separate legal entity. Hence, the death, insolvency, retirement etc. of the members do not affect the existence of the co-operatives.

(iv) **Open membership**. No limit on maximum number of membership.

(v) **Tax advantage.** Unlike other forms co–operative society is exempted from income tax and surcharge on its earnings up to a certain limit. Besides, it is also exempted from stamp duty and registration fee.

(vi) **State Assistance**. The government offers a number of grants, loans and financial assistance to the co-operative societies to make their functioning more effective.

DISADVANTAGES

(i) **Lack of secrecy**. A co-operative society has to submit its annual reports and accounts with the Registrar of Co-operative Societies. Hence it becomes quite difficult for it to maintain secrecy of its business affairs.

(ii) **Lack of interest**. The paid office bearers of co-operative societies do not take interest in the functioning of societies due to the absence of profit motive (80 co-operatives become inactive and come to a grinding halt).

(iii) **Corruption.** In a way, lack of profit motive breeds fraud and corruption in management. This is reflected in mis-appropriation of funds by the officers for their personal gains.

SELECTION OF AN APPROPRIATE FORM OF OWNERSHIP STRUCTURE

While selecting the best form of ownership structure, the entrepreneur should keep the following consideration in his/her mind:

1. Nature of business

The selection of a appropriate form of business ownership depends upon, to a great extent, the nature of the proposed business itself. For example, the business that requires personal attention and skill for their success are usually organised as and propreitary concern. Business requiring pooling of funds and skills are generally run as partnership firm. For business involved in large scale production, the company form of business ownership is preferred.

2. Area of operations

If the operation of a business is confined to an area or locality only, the appropriate form of ownership will be proprietorship/partership. On the contrary, if the area of operation is widespread catering to national or international markets, the suitable form of business ownership may be company.

3. Degree of contral

In case, direct control over business operations is required, the suitable form of ownership may be proprietorship or partnership. In case direct control over business operations is not needed, the suitable form of ownership may be a company.

4. Capital requirements

If a business requires a small amount of capital, the best form of ownership may be either propriectorship or partnership. In case of huge capital requirements, the company form of ownership will be the best.

5. Duration of business

If business is proposed for a definite duration and on adhoc basis, proprietorship or partnership are better forms of business ownership. The reason is that they are easy to form and dissolve. In case, the business is to be run on permanent basis, it can be organised as company or a co-operative because they enjoy perpetual succession.

6. Extent of risk and liability

Business involves risk. If an entrepreneur is ready and capable to bear risk involved in business, he can organise his business on proprietorship or partnership. But if the entrepreneur is hesitant to bear the risk involved in business, he can go for a company where individual risk in limited.

7. Govt. regulation

If an entrepreneur doesnot like much government involvement in his business, he can select proprietorship or partnership as the form of his business ownership instead of a company or co-operative where the government rules and regulations apply more.

5 PRODUCTION/OPERATIONS MANAGEMENT

Production is the process by which goods and services are created.

It is a system composed of number of components and can be represented as

Input → Transformation Process → Output ↗ **External environment** ↘ **Internal environment**

Inputs → various resources

Transformation process → Various activities like management processes

Output → Goods and services

Internal environment – Task, tech., people, structure

External environment – Customers, competitors, suppliers, labour unions, stock holders, government agencies etc.

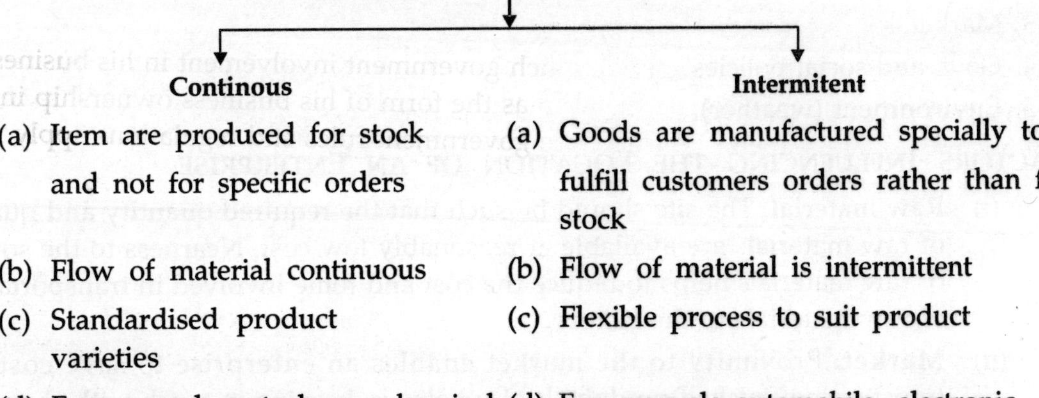

Types of Manufacturing System

Continous	**Intermitent**
(a) Item are produced for stock and not for specific orders	(a) Goods are manufactured specially to fulfill customers orders rather than for stock
(b) Flow of material continuous	(b) Flow of material is intermittent
(c) Standardised product varieties	(c) Flexible process to suit product
(d) For example petroleum, chemical, sugar industries etc.	(d) For example automobile, electronic goods, hospitals etc.

(e) Types – Mass production and Process production	(e) Types – Job production and Batch production.
(f) Regular use of machines	(f) Irregular use of machines

Plant location. Location of the industry is an important factor influencing the profitability of an enterprise. No firm can prosper unless it is situated at a place chosen from the view-point of maximum possible efficiency of operations.

Locational analysis. It is the dynamic process of analyzing and comparing the appropriateness or otherwise of alternative sites with the aim of selecting the best site for a given enterprise. It consists of the following:

(a) **Trade area analysis.** It is an analysis of the geographic area that provides continued customer to the organisation. Convenience and accessibility to the trade area from alternative sites need to be analyzed.

(b) **Demographic analysis.** It involves study of population in the area in terms of total population, age composition, per capita income, education level, occupational struc. etc

(c) **Competitive analysis.** It helps to judge the nature, location, size and quality of competition in a given trade area.

(d) **Site economics.** It is necessary to judge and compare the costs of establishment and operation at various sites under condieration. Establishment costs depend on land prices utilities etc. Operating costs include expenses on materials freight, wages and salaries, water, fuel etc.

FACTORS INFLUENCING LOCATION DECISION

1. Availability of raw materials.
2. Availability of labor.
3. Market.
4. Govt. and social policies.
5. Environment (weather).

FACTORS INFLUENCING THE LOCATION OF AN ENTERPRISE

(i) **Raw material.** The site should be such that the required quantity and quality of raw materials are available at reasonably low cost. Nearness to the source of raw materials helps to reduce the cost and tome involved in transportation of raw materials to the factory.

(ii) **Market.** Proximity to the market enables an enterprise to save costs of transporting finished product. It also helps in keeping in touch with changing market condition and in supplying quick service to customers.

(iii) **Labor.** Availability of required quality of labor is another important consideration in location. Quantity and quality of labor both should be considered.

(iv) **Government policy.** In order to achieve balanced regional development, the government offers several incentives and concession to entrepreneurs who locate their units in backward or rural areas.

(v) **Infrastructure.** Adequate and dependable transport, communication, powers, water and banking facilities are necessary for the success and growth of an industry. These should also be taken into comideration before selecting any location.

(vi) **Local laws and regulation**. In some states, antipollution laws prohibit location of polluting industries in specified areas. High local tax rates may discourage industries within some areas. Attitude of local people towards the industry should also be comidered.

PLANT LAYOUT

Plant layout refers to the arrangement of physical facilities such as machines, equipment, furniture etc. within the factory building. Prefer layout is essential for efficient manufacturing at low cost. Once the facilities are laid out, it is very difficult and costly to change the layout. A good layout will offer the following benefits.

(a) Increase in productivity.

(b) Optimum utilization of floor and other areas of operation.

(c) Effective supervision and control over industrial activities.

(d) Improvement in working environemnt.

(e) Economy in material handling.

TYPES OF LAYOUT (FOR MANUFACTURING UNITS)

These are two main types of plant layout

(a) **Product layout or line layout**

In this layout machines and equipment are arranged in a sequence required to produce a specific product. The raw materials enter the production process at one end and come out as finished product from the other end.

Raw material for product A → Drill → Grinder → Welding → Assembly → **Output**

ADVANTAGE

This layout ensures a smooth flow of materials thereby minimising work in process. It also ensures job specialisation and better utilization of floor space. It simplifies control. But it is very expensive.

DISADVANTAGE

Because of considerable duplication of machine. It is inflexible as breakdown of one machine can disrupt the entire production process.

This type is applicable to rigid flow, high volume, continuous production operation, e.g., automobile assembly plants, oil refineries etc.

(b) **Process layout (or functional layout)**

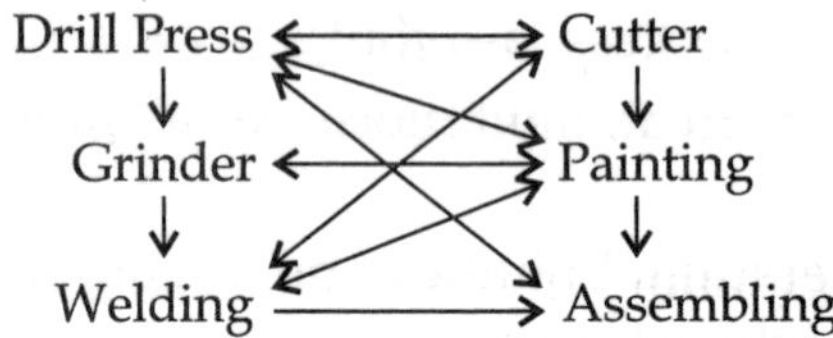

In this type of layout machines of similar type are arranged together at one place. For example, all grinding machines are placed in the grinding department. So, workers and equipments are grouped according to the general function. They perform, without regard to any particular product. These layouts are appropriate when production runs are short, when demand shows considerable variation and the costs of holding finished goods inventory are high or when the product is customized.

ADVANTAGES

(1) Flexible for doing custom work.

(2) Promotes job satisfaction by offering employees diverse and challenging tasks.

(3) More effective supervision is possible.

(4) Reduces capital investment by avoiding duplication of machines.

DISADVANTAGES

(1) Material handling costs are high.

(2) Considerable work in process.

(3) More skilled labor needed.

(4) More complex production control.

(c) **Fixed position layout**

In this raw materials do not move down a line but rather due to the weight, size or bulk of the final product, they are assembled in one spot. So workers and equipments go to the material rather than having one material flow down a line to them, e.g., aircraft assembly plants and shipyards.

FACTORS INFLUENCING LAYOUT

(1) **Factory building**. Nature and size of building, space availability within the building.

(2) **Nature of product**. Custom made or unifrom product, product design and quality standards.

(3) **Type of production process.** Technique used, types of material handles, number of operations involved.

(4) **Ergonomic considerations.** To ensure worker safety, avoid unneccessary injuries and accidents and to increase productivity.

(5) **Type of machines**. General purpose machines (product layout) or special purpose machines (process la→yout).

(6) **Plant environment.** Heat, light, noise, ventilation and other aspects should be duly considered.

(7) **Economic consideration.** Volume of production, costs of material and machines length of permissible delay etc.

RETAILERS LAYOUT/SERVICE LAYOUT

(1) **The grid layout.** A formal arrangement of displays arranged in a rectangular fashion so that asiles are parallel.

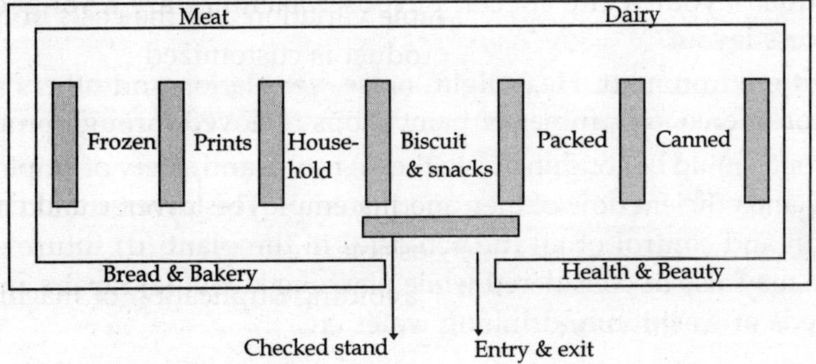

In this layout the available selling space most efficiently creates a neat, organised environment and facilities shopping by standardizing the location of items.

(2) **Free form layout**. An informal arrangement of displays of various shapes and sizes. Its primary advantage is the ralaxed, friendly shopping atmosphere it creates, which encourage customers to shop longer and increase the number of impulse purchaser.

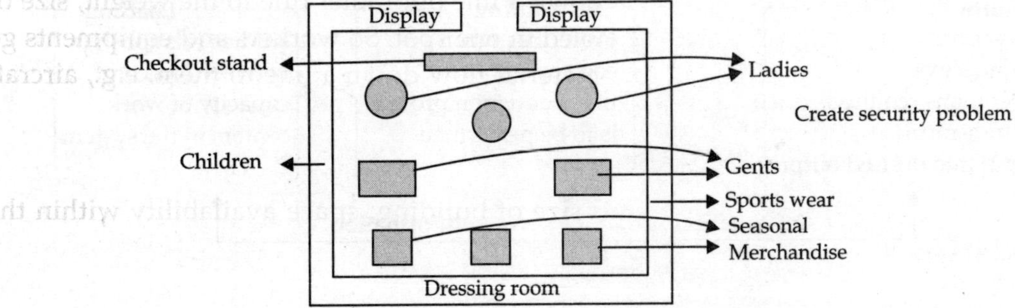

(3) **Boutique layout**. An arrangement that divides a store into a series of individual shopping areas, each with its own theme, have informal layout and create a unique shopping environment for customers. Small departmental store sometime uses this layout.

Mens | Sports | Kids
Entry
Jewellery Box | Shoes & Bags
Exit
Women | Home furnishing | Cosmetics

FACTORS INFLUENCING LAYOUT

(i) **Factory building**. Nature and size of building determines the floor space available for layout.

(ii) **Nature of product.** Job orders or assembly line industry.

(iii) **Type of machinery**. General purpose machines are often arranged as per product layout while special purpose machines are arranged according to process layout.

(iv) **Plant environment**. Heat, light, noise, ventilation and others aspects should be considered, e.g., fumes of paint shops removed through proper ventilation.

Thus layout should be conduncive to the (a) health and safety of employees. It should (b) ensure free and efficient flow of men and materials. The layout should permit effective (c) supervision and control of all the activities in the plant (d) future expansion and diversification may also be considered while planning layout (e) repairs and maintenance (f) human needs of washroom, drinking water etc.

PRODUCTION PLANNING

Concerned with planning the details of the methods required to perform each operation.

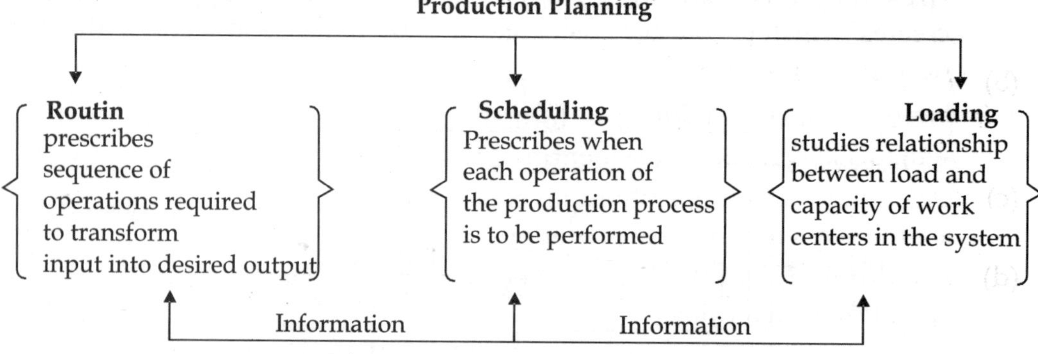

OBJECTIVES

(i) Systematic co-ordination and regulation of various activities.

(ii) Determination of raw materials, machines equipment etc. and other inputs.

(iii) Anticipation of business changes and reacting to them in proper manner.

(iv) To have optimum use of the resource with optimum cost and time.

(v) To provide alternative production strategies in the case of emergencies.

PROCEDURE FOR PRODUCTION PLANNING

The fundamental objective of production plannning is the maximum utilization of plant capacity in most economical manner.

There are three procedures of production planning:

1. Routing

Prescribes the sequence of operations required to transorm inputs into derived output. (Routing indcludes the planning that where and by whom the work shall be done).

DEFINITION

Routing means determination of path or route over which each piece is to travel in being tranformed from raw material into finished product.

Where one sinlge product or part is manufactured by a fixed set of machines, the job of routing becomes mechanical. In continious management systems with fixed line layout, it needs no managerial effort for routing. But in intermittent type of systems routing is a complex task. Routing also prescribes the amount of material, types of equipment and machines and the number of skilled and unskilled workers required to perform a particular job or operation.

ROUTING CONSISTS OF FOLLOWING STEPS

(a) The product is fabricated into sub–components to decide which components can be produced inside the plant and which parts are to be purchased from outside, i.e., to manufacture or to buy.

(b) Determine the requirement of inputs i.e. material, labor etc. The production process is then outlined in the form of drawing as a route sheet using different symbols and notation for identification.

(c) Determine various operations involved in the transformation process and then list the sequence of these operations on the route sheet.

(d) The duration and the nature of equipment and machine required for each operation is determined.

(e) The economic lot size of production order quantity is calculated.

(f) The various types of proformas to record the details of production process at different stages of production are also designed.

2. Scheduling

Scheduling is the process of prescribing 'when' each operation in a production process is to be executed. It involves designing the time table of manufacturing activities indicating the time required for the production of units at each stage

Definition. "Scheduling involves establsihing the amount of work to be done and the time when each element of the work will start".

Objectives of scheduling. The fundamental objective of scheduling is to arrange the work of the production unit in such a way that

(i) Item are delivered on due date and

(ii) Production cost is minimum.

CLASSIFICATION OF SCHEDULES

(a) **Operation schedule.** It determines the total time required to do a piece of work with a given machine or process. It indicates the time required to perform as well as other details of type of material, machines labor etc. required for each and every operation.

(b) **Master schedule.** It is a list showing how many of each item to make in each period of time in futute. These are usually changed as time moves along in response to charge in conditions. Here on the basis of sales forecast and levelling of production, the quantities to be produced are determined.

(c) **Sequential scheduling.** Here the problem is to define a sequence for a multi product plant which pass through a numbers of department. If the sequence is varied in each department the number of sequences will increase and there is no known technique to identify the optimum sequence ever assuming that the optimum can be explicitly defined.

SCHEDULING DEVICES

Gantt charts. These charts portrays planned production and actual performance over a period of time for any or all of the factors that require planning and control. It is a regular chart divided by parallel, horizontal and vertical lines.

3. Loading

It is defined as the study of the relationship between load and capacity at the places where work is done. Loading and scheduling are designed to assist in the efficient and systematic planning of work. Loading provides a complete and correct information about the number of machines available and their operating characteristics such as speed, capacity, capability etc. This information can be used to calculate the difference between work load and actual capacity and then to determine whether customer's order can be completed on due date or not.

OBJECTIVES OF LOADING

(a) To plan new work order on the basis of space capacity available.
(b) To balance the work load in a plant.
(c) To maintain the delivery promises.
(d) To check the feasibility of production programmes.

PRODUCTION CONTROL

Definision. It is a scientific procedure to regulate an orderly flow of material and co-ordinate various productions operations to accomplish the objective of producing desired item in right quantity and quality at the required time by the best and the cheapest method.

OBJECTIVES OF PRODUCTION CONTROL

(i) To see resources are used in best possible manner.
(ii) Minimise cost of production and maintain delivery date
(iii) Proper co-ordination of the operations of various sections/departments responsible for production.
(iv) To ensure regular and timely supply of raw material.
(v) To perform inspection of semi-finished and finished goods.

FACTORS DETERMINING PRODUCTION CONTROL OPERATION

1. Size/magnitude of operation (large/small).
2. Type of production (continuous/intermittent).
3. Type of product/Nature of product.

TECHNIQUES OF PRODUCTION CONTROL

Production control ensures regular and smooth flow of material and co-ordinates different manufacturing operations through the method of — programming ordering, dispatching, progressing and inventory control.

1. Programming

Production programming regulates the supply of finished product in described amount at the due date in accordance with the production plan. In production programming decisions are taken w.r.t. nature of the product to the manufactured, amount of quantities to be produced and when to produce.

2. Ordering

It breaks down the requirements for products to be completed at specific times into orders for materials and processed parts and attempts do so in such a way that they are available when needed. Information needed for ordering is requirement quantity and available quantity to get order quantity.

3. Dispatching

It is the routine of setting production activities in motion through the release of order and instruction in accordance with previously planned times and sequence given in route sheets and schedule charts.

The decision of assigning various jobs to different machines is known as dispatching.

FUNCTIONS OF DISPATCHING

(i) To check immediate availability of materials.
(ii) Ensure that all production and inspection aids we available for use.
(iii) Assign the work to definite machines, men.
(iv) Issue necessary material, tools etc. for use.
(v) To issue production order note stating the start and finish times.
(vi) Maintain all production records viz. time lost in production and causes of delay: machine breakdown, material delay, absenterism etc.

4. Progressing/follow up

It is ascertaining from time to time that the production operations are progressing according to the plan. Follow up can be done at three stages — for materials, work in progress and/end stage during assembly. It discovers factors causing delays which may be scheduled beyond the capacity of the machine, underestimating of material, tools and manpower, errors in processing and inspection etc.

This is the function by which one can give early warning when actual production deviates from planned production and thus makes it possible to take corrective action.

Progressing uses machine load charts, production schedule and inspection reports etc. and does following steps:

(i) Recording actual production.
(ii) Compare it with planned production.
(iii) Measure the variability in production.
(iv) Corrective action and reporting the matter to higher authority.

5. Inventory control

Its main aim is to observe the stock investment and to ensure it lies within the limits which the organisation can afford.

ADVANTAGES OF PRODUCTION CONTROL

1. It ensures quality and quantity of the product
2. Minimize the chances of product rejection by customer.
3. Guarantees timely supply of goods in the market.

Functions of planning and control in production management are closely related with each other. Planning concerns with the formulation of production straegies and targets for the enterprise whereas control is related to actual implementation and execution of planned objectives. Production planning determines the operations required to manufacture same product and control regulates and supervises these operation.

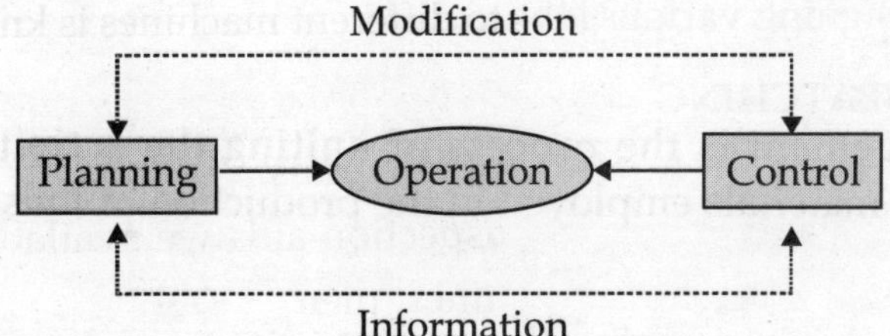

Fig. Relation between operations, planning and control

6 MATERIALS MANAGEMENT

Materials management is the process of uniting the activities involved in the acquisition and use of materials employed in the production of finished goods products.

DEFINITION

1. "Materials management is controlling the kind, amount, location, movement and timing of various commodities used in production by the organisations".
2. Material management deals with controlling and regulating, the flow of material in relation to changes in variables like demand, prices, availability, quality, delivery etc.

Various functions of materials management are :

1. Planning and programming for materials purchase.
2. Stores and stock control.
3. Receiving and issue of the material.
4. Transportation of material (handling of the material).
5. Value engineering and value analysis (value of an item can be defined as the ratio of its worth to its cost).
6. Disposal of scrap and surplus materials.

FUNDAMENTAL OBJECTIVES

Material management contributes to survival and profits of an organisation by providing adequate supply of materials at the lowest possible costs. The fundamental objectives can be:

1. Material selection. Correct specification of material and components is determined. Also the material requirement in agreement with sales programme are assessed. This can be done by analysing the requirition order of the buying department with this standardisation one many have lower cost and the task of procurement, replacement etc., may be easier.

2. Low operating costs. Material management should keep the operating costs low and increase the profits without making only concession in quality.

3. Issue material upon receipt of appropriate authority, i.e., to supply regular uninterrupted supply of raw materials to ensure continuity of production.

4. To minimize storage and stock control costs.

DUTIES OF MATERIALS MANAGER

Material management embraces all functions concerned with ordering, storage and movement of materials, i.e., purchasing, production control stores, traffic and physical distribution. These are:

1. Purchasing

Purchasing dept buys materials in amount is authorised by requisitions receiving from the production control and storer department. Its main operations are:

(a) Selection of suppliers and issue of purchase order.

(b) To expedite delivery of material from the suppliers.

(c) Acting as a liasion between suppliers and other depts of the organisation.

(d) To look for new products, materials and suppliers that can contribute to company's profits.

2. Production control. This is done by

(a) Determining requirements of materials and parts to be purchased and manufactured.

(b) Schedules production and purchasing processes of parts and materials.

(c) Issues work order to manufacturing department and purchase order to suppliers.

3. Inventary and stores control

It keeps detailed and up-to-date record of inventory, on order status and potential demand for each production part and material. It is also responsible for non-productive stores like office supplies, perishable goods etc.

4. Traffic

It controls inbound shipments of purchased material and outbound shipment of finished goods to consumers. This is done by

(a) Selection of carriers

(b) Auditing invoice from carriers and filing claims for refund in case of excess charges or damaged shipments

(c) Developing techniques to reduce transportation costs.

5. Physical distribution

Finished goods are moved from the production line to the warehouse and finally to the customer.

INVENTORY COSTS

In operating an inventory system mangers should consider only those costs that vary directly with the operating doctrine in deciding when and how much to recorder; costs independent of the operating doctrine are irrelevant. Basically following types of relevant costs are these (these often combine in one way or another).

1. Cost of item

The cost, or value of the item is usually its purchase price, the amount paid to the supplies for the item. In some cases, however, transportation, receiving, or inspection costs, for example, may be included as part of the cost of the item. If the cost of item per unit is constant for all quantities ordered, the total cost of items purchased during the planning horizon is irrelevant. If the unit cost varies with the quantity ordered, a price reduction called quantity discount, this cost is relevant.

If the facility manufactures the item, the cost of the item is its direct manufacturing cost.

2. Procurement costs

Procurement costs are the costs of placing a purchase order, or the set up costs if the item is manufactured at the facility. These costs vary directly with each purchase order placed. Procurement costs include costs of postage, telephone calls to the vendor, labor costs in purchasing and accounting, receiving costs, computer time for record keeping and purchase order supplies.

3. Carrying (holding) costs

Carrying or holding costs are the costs of maintaining the inventory warehouse and protecting the inventoried, items. Typical costs are insurance, security, warehouse, rental, heat, lights, taxes and losses due to pilferage, or breakage. The cost of typing up capital in inventory is also considered a carrying cost.

4. Stock out costs

Stock out costs, associated with demand when stocks have been depleted, take the form of lost sales or back order costs. When sales are lost because of stock outs, the firm loses both the profit margin on unmade sales and its customer's good will. If customer take their business elsewhere, future profit margins may also be lost.

When customers agree to come back after inventories have been replenished, they make back orders. Back order costs include loss of good will and money paid to recorder goods and notify customer when goods arrive.

5. Cost of operating the information processing system

Whether by hand or by computer, someone must update records as stock levels change. For systems in which inventory levels are not recorded daily, the cost is primarily incurred in obtaining accurate physical counts of inventories, frequently. These operating costs are more fixed than variable over a wide quantity range. (These costs are mainly irrelevant because they are fixed.)

COST TRADE OFFS

The objective of inventory control is to find the minimum cost operating doctrine over some planning horizon. Using a one year planning horizon, the control costs can be expressed in a general equalation

Total annual relevant costs	= Cost of the items	+ Procurement	+ Carrying cost	+ Stock out cost
			• Cycle stocks	• Cost sales
			• Buffer stocks	• Back order

Each cost in the equation can be expressed in terms of order, quality and recorder point for a given inventory situation. The solution method is then to minimise the total cost. This can be accomplished graphically; by tabular analysis using trial and error or by using calulus, the most accurate method — operation researches have developed a wide range of optimal formulas, using calculus, which vary with changes in the actual inventory situation (graphicaly, minimising total costs means cost trade offs).

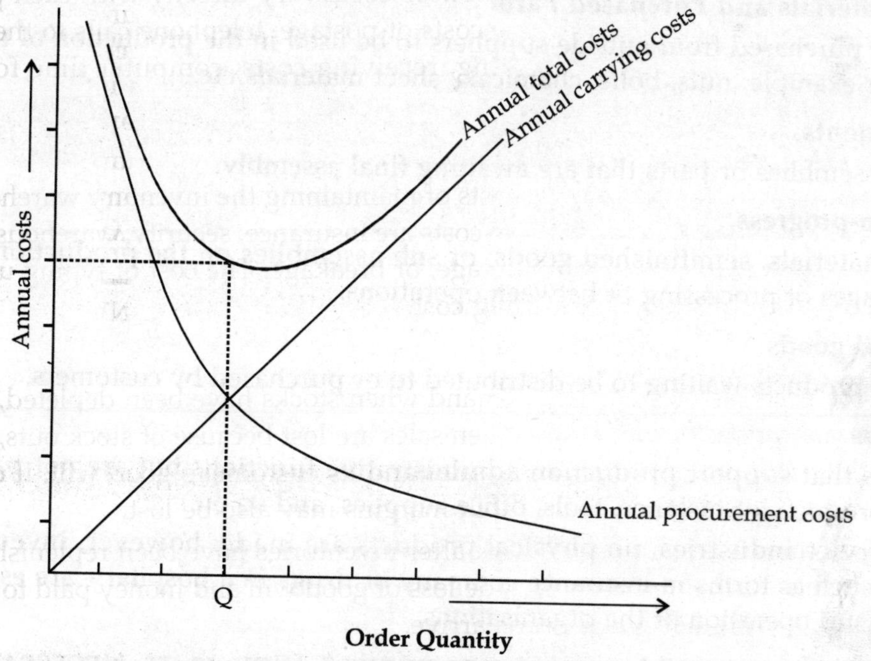

Fig. Cost trade offs in inventory control
(Q is the optimal order quantity or economic order quantity)

In above figure for a simple model in which cost of item and cost of stockout are irrelevant, the trade off is only between only two costs procurement and carrying costs. Note that annual carrying costs increase with larger value of order quantity Q. (Likewise where Q is large, fewer orders must be placed during the year so that the annual procurement cost decreases). There is a cost trade off between the two. If we add the costs graphically we obtain a total cost curve. The optimal orders quantity Q is the point at which annual total cost is minimum.

INVENTORY CONTROL (MATERIAL CONTROL)

Inventory is stores of goods and stocks. In manufacturing, items in inventory are called stock keeping items, held at a stock (storage) point. Stock keeping items usually are raw materials, work-in-progress, finished products supplies etc.

Inventory control is activities that maintain stock keeping items at desired levels. In manufacturing, since the focus is on a physical product, inventory control focuses on materials control. In the service sector, since the focus is on a service (often consumed as generated), inventory focuses less on materials and more on supplies. For service organisations that are not highly labor-intensive, inventories assume more importance. Transit systems maintain inventories of equipment and replacement parts.

FIVE TYPES OF INVENTORY

Several types of inventory are carried out. These are:

1. Raw Materials and Purchased Parts

Items purchased from outside suppliers to be used in the production of the firm's output, for example, nuts, bolts, chemicals, sheet materials etc.

2. Components

Subassemblies or parts that are awaiting final assembly.

3. Work-in-progress

All materials, semifinished goods, or sub-assemblies on the production floor in various stages of processing or between operations.

4. Finished goods

Final products waiting to be distributed to or purchased by customers.

5. Supplies

Items that support production administrative functions but are not part of the finished product; for instance, tools, office supplies, and so on.

In service industries, no physical products are made; however, inventories of supplies, such as forms in insurance company or drugs in a hospital – are essential to the successful operation of the organisations.

NEED FOR CARRYING/MAKING INVENTORIES? WHY IS IT NECESSARY?

There are four principal reasons as to why an organisation carries inventory. These are

1. It is very rarely possible to predict sales levels and production times accurately. Thus fluctuation inventories, most often safety stock, are maintained in orders to minimize the effect of such variations.
2. Many items have high seasonal demand. It might be impossible to produce enough during a short selling season due to limited production capacity. Anticipation inventories are filled up during the off season in order to meet the estimated demand.
3. Third reason for maintaining inventory is to take advantage of economics of scale in production and purchasing. The purchase of large lots often brings savings through quantity discounts and truckload-discount transportation rates, though the entire quantity is not required all at once.
4. A significant amount of stock is usually in transit line. Various stages in the logistics systems for e.g., the shipment goods from factories to regional warehouses by truck or rail may take several days or week. This pipeline inventory cannot be used until it reaches its distination.

Other Primary Reason for Carrying Inventory

1. Physical impossibility of getting right amount of stock at right time of need.
2. Economical impracticality of getting right amount of stock at exact time of need.

Inventory System

Q/R Inventory system (Also called Continuous Review System)

One way to establish an inventory system is to keep count of every item issued from inventory and place an order for more stock when inventories dwindle to a predetermined level, the recorder point (i.e., the time to recorder). The recorder quantity, also called the economic order quantity, is fixed in size (volume), size having been predetermined.

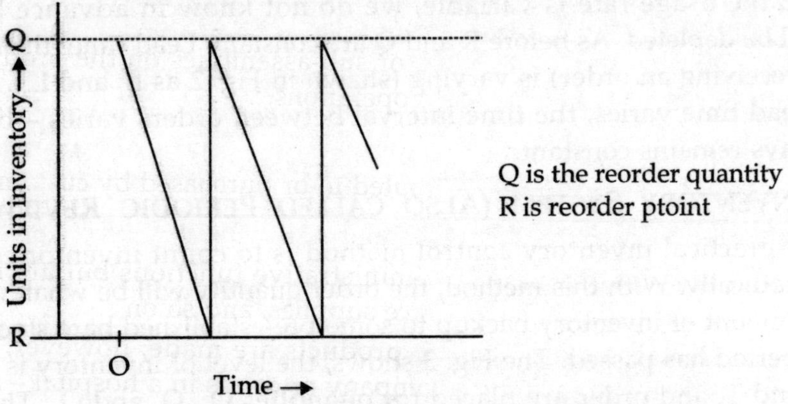

Fig. 1. Q/R Inventory system: Constant usage rate (R is the records point and Q the order quantity)

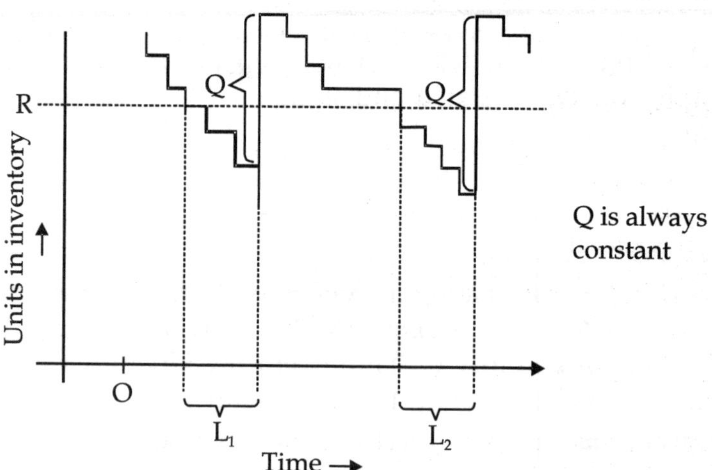

Fig. 2. Q/R Inventory system: Variable usage rate
(R is the recorder point, Q the order quantity and L is the lead time)

Figs. 1 and 2 illustrate two types of Q/R inventory systems. For fig.1 the demand for inventories, also called usage rate, is known and constant. Replenishment inventories are assumed to be received at the stock point the moment they have been ordered. Procurement lead time is zero. In this case, there is no need to carry buffer stocks. As time goes by inventory is steadily depleted until a level of R is reached (R is the reorder point), and then an order for Q units is placed. These units arrive at the instant they are ordered. As delivery is instantaneous and the demand for the inventory item is known for certain the R is set at zero units. (So lead time is zero here).

In a Q/R system, both the reorder quantity and the reorder point are fixed. Thus in Fig. 1 both are constant.

In Fig. 2 the usage rate is variable, we do not know in advance how rapidly inventory will be depleted. As before R and Q are constant. Lead time (the time taken in placing and receiving an order) is varying (shawn in Fig. 2 as L_1 and L_2). When either demand or lead time varies, the time interval between orders varies – but the order quantity always remains constant.

PERIODIC INVENTORY SYSTEM (ALSO CALLED PERIODIC REVIEW SYSTEM)

Another practical inventory control method is to count inventories at set time intervals, periodically. With this method, the order quantity will be whatever is needed to bring the amount of inventory backup to some pre-established bare stock level, after a fixed time period has passed. The Fig. 3 shows, the level of inventory is examined at times T_1, T_2 and T_3 and order are placed for quantities Q_1, Q_2 and Q_3. The base stock level and the time T between orders are set by operations management and comprise the inventory system's is operating doctrine.

The Fig. 3 is showing constant demand within any one review period and zero lead time. These conditions could be related and still show the periodic inventory system concepts to be retained.

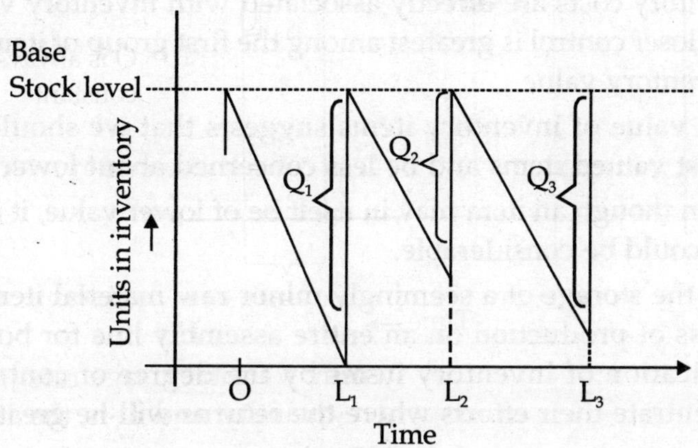

Fig. 3 Peroidic inventory system

(T is the time between and Q_1 the order quantities)

"ABC" Classification of Inventory Items

The concept of ABC Inventory Analysis was first proposed by H.F. Dickie in the early 1950 at GE for studying inventories consisting of a large number of different items. The technique is a very valuable management tool for identifying and controlling important inventory items.

For example, Fig. 4 shows a fairly typical relationship between the percentage of inventory items and the percentage of inventory's total rupee value.

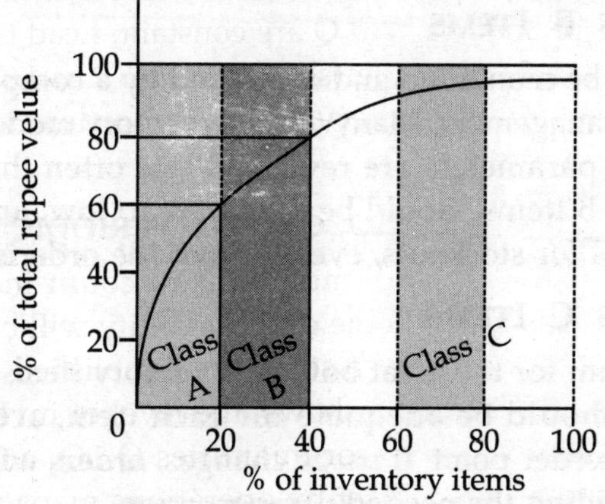

Fig. 4. ABC classification of inventory items.

The fig. 4 shows that 20% of the items account for 60% of the inventory's total Rs. value. The second 20% of the items account for 20% of the value percentage and finally, the greatest percentage of items i.e., 60% accounts for only 20% of total inventory value.

Because inventory costs are directly associated with inventory value, the potential cost savings from closer control is greatest among the first group of items, which accounts for most of the inventory value.

The different value of inventory items suggests that we should concentrate our attention on highest valued items and be less concerned about lower valued items.

Secondly, even though an item may in itself be of lower value, it is possible that the cost of a stockout could be considerable.

For example, the storage of a seemingly minor raw material item could cause idle labor costs and loss of production on an entire assembly line for both the preceeding reasons. A classification of inventory items by the degree of control needed allows managers to concentrate their efforts where the returns will he greatest.

CONTROL FOR CLASS A ITEMS

Close control is required for inventory items that have high stockout costs and those item that account for a large fraction of the total inventory value. The closest control might be reserved for raw materials that are used continuously in extremly high volume. Purchasing agents may arrange contracts with vendors for the continuous supply of these materials at rates that match usage rates. Changes in the rate of flow are made periodically as demand and inventory position changes. Minimum supplies are maintained to guard against demand fluctuations and possible interruptions of supply.

For the balance of Class A items, periodic ordering, perhaps on a weekly basis, provides the necessary close surveillance over inventory levels.

CONTROL FOR CLASS B ITEMS

These items should be monitored and controlled by a computer based system, with periodic review by the management. Many of the inventory models are relevant for these items. However, model parameters are reviewed less often than with Class A items. Stockout costs for Class B items should be moderate to low, and buffer stocks should provide adequate control for stockouts, even though the ordering occurs less often.

CONTROL FOR CLASS C ITEMS

Class C items account for the great bulk of inventory items and carefully designed but rountine controls should be adequate for each item, action is triggered when inventories fall to the recorder point. If usage changes, orders will be triggered earlier or later than average, providing the needed compensation.

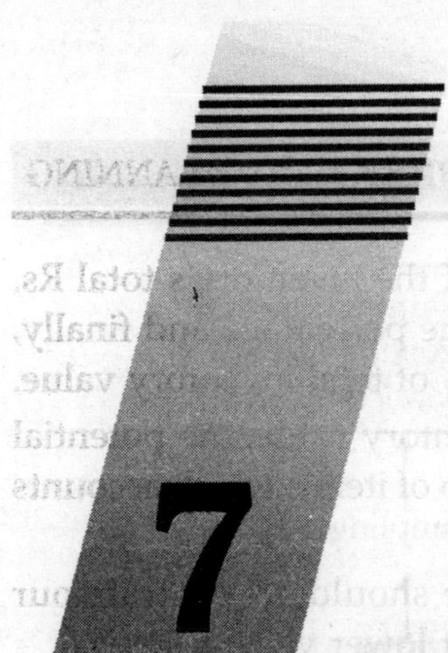

7 QUALITY CONTROL

No business small or large can be successful without providing product of right quantity to customers. In order to maintain quality, regular control over raw materials, production process and finished product it essential. Such control is called quality control.

DEFINITION

The systematic control of all variables influencing the quality of the final product are called quality control. It is a system by which products are made to measure upto the specifications determined from customer's requirement and engineering capabilities.

Advantages:

1. Helps to reduce cost
2. Facilitates standardisation
3. Improves brand image of the enterprise
4. Enables the manufactures to comply with quality standards prescribed by the government.

Measuring Quality (Quality Control). Quality control takes place at many points in a production system

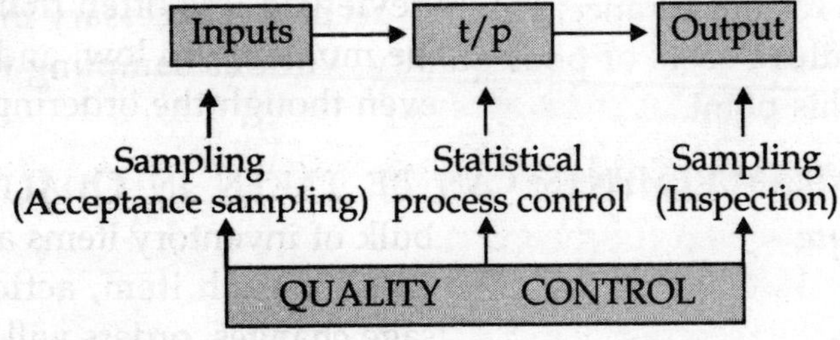

MEASURING QUALITY/QUALITY CONTROL

Quality control inspection and measurement take place at many points in a production systems. See Fig.1.

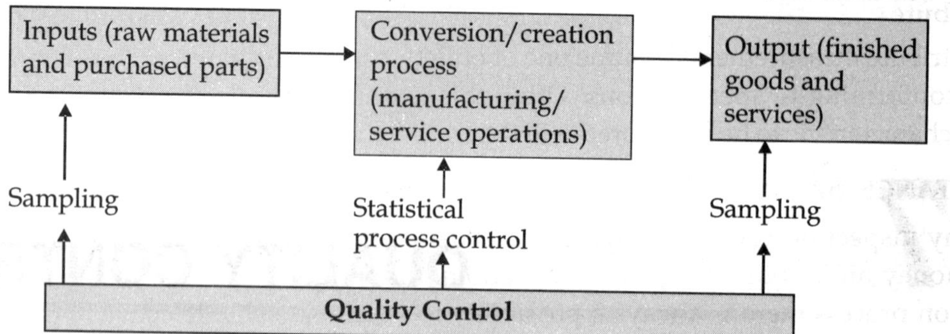

Fig. 1. The use of quality control in production

Quality control inspection and measurement take place at many points in a production system. These are:

1. The inspection of raw materials and purchased parts is usually part of the receiving operation. The purpose of such an inspection task is to determine whether or not incoming parts are of acceptable quality to be used in production, as specified by the standards developed during the product design effort. Inspection to make an accept-or-reject decision at receiving can encourage higher quality in manufacturing, since the vendor knows that poor-quality lots will be returned at his or her expense. The quality control technique that is used is called acceptance sampling.
2. Between various stages of a production process, work in process is inspected to uncover possible problems in machinery or human performance. As tools wear out, for instance, they need to be replaced in order to manufacture the item properly. Therefore, it is necessary to examine the production output over time to see if any changes have occurred. Statistical process control is widely used technique for monitoring work-in-process.
3. Finally, after the finished product is complete, as inspection is usually performed. This may be a mechanical or electronic test for performance or a visual inspection for appearance. Final inspection is necessary in order to minimize internal failure costs of poor quality. Various sampling techniques are also useful at this point.

Two Types of Measurements can be taken in Quality Control

Variable or Attribute

1. Variable

A variable measurement is a measurement of a physical quantity such as diameter, length, weight or any characteristic that takes on continuous values. This kind of measurement is generally performed with some type of instrument.

2. Attribute

Attribute measurements assume one of only two possible values, such as conforming or not conforming to specifications. Often this is done through visual inspection. The quality characteristic to be monitored will determine the type of measurement to be taken.

ACCEPTANCE SAMPLING OR SAMPLING INSPECTION STATISTICAL SAMPLING

Any inspection procedure involving 100% inspection needs huge expenditure of time, money and labor. Also due to boredom and jatigue, involved in the repetitive inspection process there is always a possibility to overlook some defective item even by most competent and efficient inspectors. Therefore 100% inspection cannot be planned.

The alternative is statistical sampling inspection methods. The purpose of sampling inspection is to estimate the quality of an entire lot by inspecting only a small portion of it. In a statistical sense sampling inspection is simply a test of the hypothesis that a lot of acceptable quality versus the alternative hypothesis that the lot is not acceptable.

The advantages of sampling are:

(a) It is less costly – in term of time and cost of inspection.

(b) Greater efficiency – as it require less time, and boredom compared to the 100% inspection, hence efficiency increases.

(c) There is less handling and hence less chance of damage.

The disadvantages of sampling are:

1. The risk of accepting poor quality lots.
2. Rejecting good-quality lots.
3. Significant planning and documentation is required.

In statistical sampling mainly two types of errors can the made = Type I and Type II errors.

Type I error is denoted by a and it is called as producer's risk.

Type II error is denoted by b and is called consumer's risk.

Producer's risk refer to the probability of rejecting of a good lot. Consumer's risk refer to the probability of accepting a bad lot.

VARIOUS SAMPLING PLANS

The programme of acceptance sampling depends on the method of selecting the sample and the acceptance level of defectives. There are a number of sampling schemes known as sampling plans. This choice depends upon the nature of the manufacturing system and the degree of consumer and producer's risks which one wants to cover. Some of the sampling schemes also–

1. Single sampling plan

Here a single sample of size 'n' is drawn from a lot of size 'N' and lot is accepted if the number of defectives in the lot (d) is less than the specification (c), i.e., A sample of size 'n' is drawn and the items of the sample are inspected. Let the number of defectives in the sample be 'd'. If

(a) $d \leq c$, the lot is accepted and the defective items i.e., d are replaced.

(b) If $d > c$, the lot is rejected and then the entries lot is inspected and the defective items are replaced.

2. Double sampling plan

This type of scheme is more economical than single sampling scheme when the quality of incoming goods in high. Here sample is drawn in two stages. The second sample is drawn when clear cut decision cannot be drawn from the first sample. Let C_1 and C_2 be the specified defectives in first and second samples respectively. The following are the steps in the method.

(a) Draw a sample of size n, from the lot. Inspect the item of the sample and let d_1 be the number of defective item. If $d_1 < c_1$, the lot is accepted after replacing the d_1 defective item. If the $d_1 > c_2$, the lot is rejected and all the items of the lot are inspected and defectives replaced. If $c_1 < d_1 < c_2$, go to step (b).

(b) Take another sample of size n_2 and let the number of defective items in the second sample be d_2. Thus, the total number of defective, item in a sample size $n_1 + n_2$ from the lot will now be $d = d_1 + d_2$. If d £ c_2 accept the lot after replacing defective items. If $d > c_2$ reject the lot. All the items of the lot are inspected and defective replaced.

It is experienced that lots with borderline defective items have a better opportunity of being accepted in double sampling scheme. But the perunit inspection cost in double sampling is found to be higher in single sampling scheme.

(c) **Sequential sampling plan.** This plan is simply as extension of double sampling plan. At each stage of sampling, the cumulated results are analysed to take a decision of accepting or rejecting a lot. If at any stage no final decision can be taken, then another sample is drawn to take further decision. This scheme helps in reducing the size of inspection to maintain a given level of protection.

The preference of any sampling scheme/plan mainly depends on the degree of accuracy desired by the organisation as well as the resources available for production.

Uses of acceptance sampling

1. Reduction in the cost and time associated with inspection.
2. Inspection process is less complicated and can be carried out more sincerely.
3. Production cost is reduced due to reduction of defective item.

STATISTICAL QUALITY CONTROL

This is applied by taking samples and drawing conclusions by means of some mathematical analysis. It is known that variation in the quality of the product is an inherent characteristic of a manufacturing system. Irrespective of all possible precaution and quality measures there are always a large number of random disturbances responsible for derivation in the quality of the product from the set standards. These are of two types:

1. Chance causes

These can neither be controlled or removed. The presence of these causes in the systems is due to a multitude of reasons which are difficult to identify and uneconomical to eliminate, e.g., movement of the machine due to passing traffic, sudden changes in temperature etc.

2. Assignable causes

These causes can be identified and eliminated economically. The magnitude of variability due to these causes varies with the condition of the production process, nature of raw material, behavior of operations etc.

The reasons for the presence of assignable causes can be:

(i) Differences among the worker's performance.

(ii) Difference among machines.

(iii) Variation in material.

The chance and assignable causes combine together to lower the quality of the product. Any item which is not in accordance with the quality specification is known as defective item and is liable to be rejected by producer and consumer.

Statistical quality control is the method to as certain whether the variation in the quality of the product is due to chance causes or of due to assignable causes.

If the process is found to be statistical control when it indicates that the variation in the quality is due to chance causes only. Otherwise presence of assignable causes is detected and same corrective action is planned to improve the quality of the product.

CONTROL CHARTS ARE THE BASIS OF STATISTICAL QUALITY CONTROL TECHNIQUE

BENEFITS OF STATISTICAL QUALITY CONTROL

1. The use of statistical quality control ensures rapid and efficient inspection at a minimum cost.
2. It minimises waste by identifying the causes of excessive variability in the quality of product.

3. SQC exerts more effective pressure for quality improvement than 100% inspection.
4. Application of statistical technique further minimises and judgemental error.

CONTROL CHARTS

The concept of control charts and their use in production systems was introduced by Shswart in 1924.

Here the whole production line is divided into a number of subgroups. The basis of selecting these subgroups is such that variation in the quality of items within each subgroup is attributed due to chance causes, whereas the corresponding variation between various sub-groups can be due to assignable causes.

The following factor should be considered while selecting a subgroup:

(i) Each sub group should be as homogeneous as possible

(ii) Sample should not be taken at exactly equal intervals of time.

(iii) There must be a maximum opportunity for variation from one subgroup to another.

STATISTICAL BASIS OF CONTROL CHART

In statistics it is assumed that various characteristics observed in different areas of study are found to follow any of the Normal, Poisson or Binomial distribution. These distributions are characterized by their mean and standard deviation. In the case of production process the quality Q can be expressed in terms of some dimension viz. life of an electric bulb, diameter of rod etc. or some other measure of performance viz. colour, weight etc.

Let the whole process be divided into 'K' subgroups each containing 'n' items. Now the quality characteristic can be measured for all the items of various subgroups. The mean and standard deviation can be calculated for each subgroup.

K subgroup 'n' items	Quality characteristics for all	Find mean (M) and standard deviation (σ)

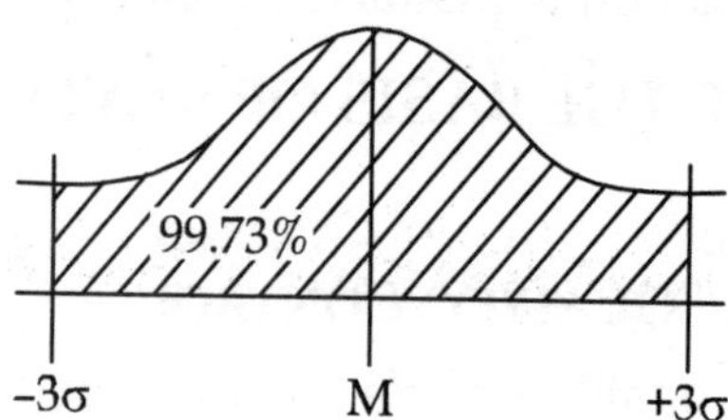

Now, (1) Statistical theory assumes that if 'M' and 's'are near mean and standard deviation of the quality characteristic over all subgroups, then the quality characteristic 'Q' will follow any of the standard distributions with mean M and standard deviation s.

(2) Also statistical theory states that for sample size to be sufficiently large, every theoretical distribution tend to a normal distribution. In a normal distribution M± s limits contains approximately 99.73% of the observations.

Similarly M ± 1.96 σ contains 95% observations.

This fundamental concept of normal distribution becomes the basis of control charts, i.e., if all the values of Q lie within M ± 3σ limits then this is an indication that assignable causes are absent and the process is said to be in control otherwise the process is said to be out of control and some remedial actions is planned.

M+3σ and M–3σ are known as upper (U.C.L.) and lower (L.C.L.) control limits respectively. The fixation of the control limits for a process is based on the assumption that the system is stable and only chance causes are present. In case assignable causes are operative in the system then quality characteristics will fall outside the two control limits.

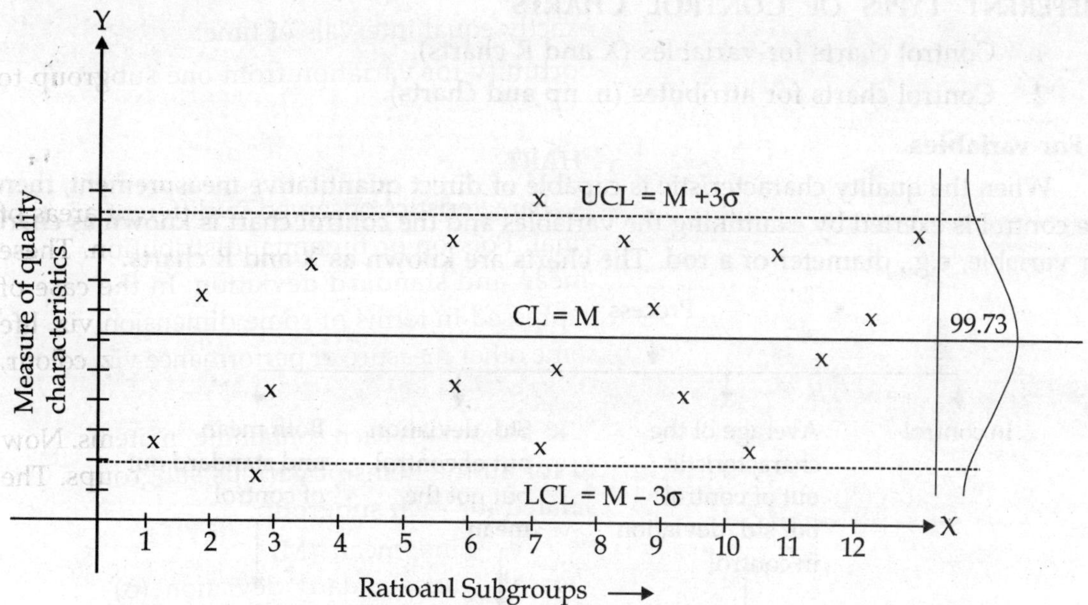

A typical control chart is shawn above. The following are its main characteristics:-

1. **Rational subgroup.** which can be taken in orders of time or sample number taken on horizontal axis (X).
2. Quality characteristic measure for each subgroup is taken on vertical axis (Y).
3. U.C.L. (M+3s) and L.C.L. (M–3s) are drawn as horizontal lines and shown by dotted lines.
4. C.L. at a distance M on Y axis is drawn between U.C.L. and L.C.L. and is represented by a dark line.

5. Points are plotted on the graph for each group and its corresponding quality characteristic.

The following interpretations can be made by the study of a control chart.

(i) If all the points in the chart lie within U.C.L. and L.C.L. then the proccess is said to be in control indicating presence of chance causes only.

(ii) If one or more points lie beyond U.C.L. and L.C.L. then the process is said to be out of control showing the presence of assignable causes and the necessity of some remedial actions.

(iii) If all points lie predominantly on one side of the central line then it is not safe to derive any conclusion about the process control.

Thus a control chart is a graphical representation of the range of enpected variability in a production process.

DIFFERENT TYPES OF CONTROL CHARTS

1. Control charts for variables (X and R charts).
2. Control charts for attributes (n, np and charts).

1. For variables

When the quality characteristic is capable of direct quantitative measurement, then the control is exerted by examining the variables and the control chart is known as chart for variable, e.g., diameter of a rod. The charts are known as X and R charts.

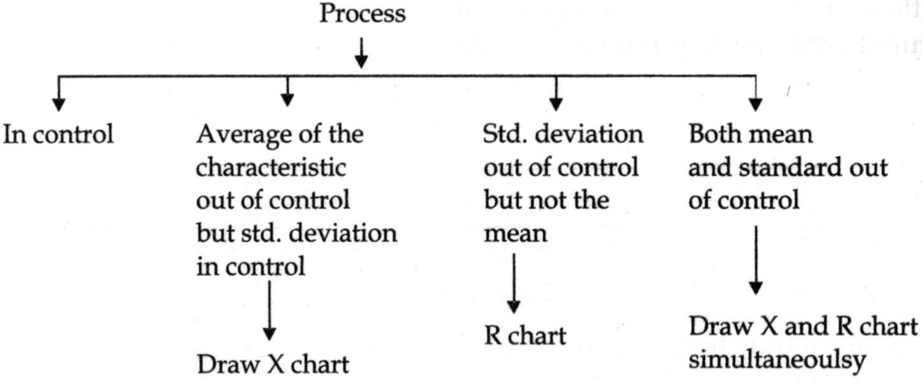

2. Control charts for attributes

If the quality characteristic is not capable of direct quantitative measurement and the items can be classified only as "good" or "bad", acceptable or not acceptable (e.g., quality of a cloth, etc.), then control is exerted by examining attributes and the corresponding chart is known as chart for attributes. (Here the quality characteristic is assumed to follow binomial or Poisson distribution).

The Charts are known as p, np and c Charts

QUALITY CONTROL IN SSI

Quality control is more essential for SSI due to labor intensive methods of production. But effective quality control in these units is difficult due to technical, financial and managerial constraints.

In India, Bureau of Indian Standards (BIS) has been doing a great service by prescribing quality standards for a large number of products. In the small sector quality control is based on:

(i) Indian standards specifications.
(ii) Quality marketing schemes.
(iii) Company standards for ancillary units.
(iv) Standards specified by purchasing agencies.

For controlling quality of products manufactured by small units, the following manuals have been published so far:

(a) Methods of statistical quality control during the production period,
(b) Manual on basic principles of lot sampling, and
(c) Sampling inspection tables.

Several state governments have also been operating marketing scheme and standards for various products of SSI. When the small units manufacture their products according to the standards set, the quality marketing centres of the Govt. stamp the 'Q' mark on their products. This is assurance for the customers that the product has been manufactured adhering to certain quality standards.

MARKETING

DEFINITION

1. Marketing is a human activity directed at satisfying needs and wants, through an exchange process.
2. Marketing consists of all those activities that direct the flow of goods and services from the producer to the consumer/user.

MARKETING IS MUCH WIDER THAN SELLING

Selling	Marketing
1. Emphasis on the product	1. Emphasises on customer's wants
2. Sales are the primary motive	2. Satisfaction of customers is primary
3. First production, then selling takes place at a profit without knowing customer's need	3. First customer's need is known and then production takes place, and then product is sold at a profit
4. Costs determines price	4. Customer determines price and price determines cost.
5. It is an activity that converts goods into cash	5. It is a function that converts the consumer needs into products.

MARKETING MIX

The modern market concept emphasies the importance of customer's preference. Marketing Mix' is the term used to describe the combination of the four inputs which constitute the core of a company's marketing system – the product, the price structure, the promotional activities and the distribution system. These are popularly known as 4 P's.

Product	Price	Place	Promotion
Features Design	Credit terms Payment period	Channels Location	Advertising Sales promotion

Brand Package Service Warranty Quality Style	Discount Price	Delivery Transport Wholeselling Relating (warehousing) Inventory control	Publicity Selling Communication

The elements of four P's are interelated, complementary and mutually supporting ingredients. Marketing Mix is used as a tool towards the customer in order to ascertain their needs, tastes and preferences etc.

Four P's	Four C's
Product	Customer need
Price	Cost to the customer
Place	Convenience
Promotion	Communication

FUNCTIONS OF MARKETING

1. Market Research
2. Product Planning and Development
3. Procurement of Resources like machines, materials etc.
4. Identification of the target groups and understanding them from all possible angles to know their taste, habit, customs etc.,
5. Product standardization
6. Branding
7. Packaging
8. Pricing
9. Distribution of products to various locations
10. Advertising
11. Selling
12. After-sale service

MARKETING INFORMATION

Adequate and up-to-date information about changing market conditions is necessary for successful marketing of products. Decisions concerning the type of product, the price policy, the channel of distribution and sales promotion can be made rightly with the help of right marketing information at the right time.

In order to collect marketing information, LSI conduct market research. SSI's are often unable to afford continuous marketing research. However, they can use personal contacts and other informal methods for collecting required information about markets.

Marketing information can be collected from the following sources:

I. Primary Source

(a) Customers

(b) Dealers

(c) Salesman

II. Secondary Source

(a) **Press.** (e.g., Economics Times and Business Today).

(b) **Govt. publications.** (Different Ministeries and departments of the Central Government and State Government publish regularly some journals, periodicals etc. Which contain very useful data relating to business e.g. Annual report on the working of public understandings; import policy; guidelines for industries etc.).

(c) **Publication of financial institutions.** The RBI, public financial institutions and commercial banks publish a lot of useful information (e.g. monthly bulletin of RBI etc.).

(d) **Publication of trade associations.** Trade associations and chambers of commerce collect and publish useful data for the benefit of their members (useful to analyse business trends in India).

(e) **Private concerns and research institutions.** Some research institutes like National Council of Applied Economic Research, Indian Institutes of Foreign Trade, etc. Conduct research studies regularly and publish data of various types. Private agencies like FICCI also publish data.

MARKET SEGMENTATION

A market consists of heterogenous customers who differ in terms of their needs, preferences and buying capacity. A different marketing approach is necessary for every customer group. Therefore it becomes necessary to divide the total market into diffrent segments or homogenous customer groups. Such division is called market segmentation.

DEFINITION

Market segmentation is the sub-dividing of a market into homogenous subsets of customers where any subset may be selected as a target market to be reached with a distinct marketing mix.

Market segmentation enables the entrepreneur to fine tune his marketing efforts so as to match the requirements of the target market as well as possible. Instead of waisting his efforts in trying to sell to all types of customers, a unit can focus its efforts on the segment most appropriate to its marketing programme.

BRANDING

It is the process of assigning a distinctive name to the product by which it is to be known and remembered. A brand may be a name, symbol, design, photograph or a combination there of that helps to differentiate a product from the competitive products. When the brand is registered under the Trade and Mercantile Marks Act, 1958, it becomes a trademark, e.g., Lux, Singer, Philips, LG, BPL are example of brands.

BENEFITS OF BRANDING

(i) It helps the consumer to identify and recognize the product.

(ii) It helps in differentiating your product from the rival products.

(iii) It is the basis of advertising and other techniques of mass selling.

(iv) Branding ensource uniform standards of quality and design to consumers.

PACKAGING

It refers to wrapping of goods before they are transported, stored or delivered to a consumer.

FUNCTIONS/ADVANTAGE OF PACKAGING

(i) **Product protection.** Package protects the products. Package prevents breakage, contamination, insect attack etc.

(ii) **Product containant.** Package means just using the space in which a product will be contained. Ordinary packing in the form of throw away containers is the example.

(iii) **Product attractiveness.** The size and shape of the package its color, printed matter on it etc., make the package attractive to look at. Psychological feeling is that a good package contains good quality in it.

(iv) **Product identification.** Packages differentiate similar products. Packaging and labelling are inseparable and are closely related to branding. Package has more significance when the product cannot be seen by the buyer, e.g., packed milk, fruit juice etc.

(v) **Effective sales tool.** A good package stimulates sales. A well designed and attractive package invites customers.

PRICING POLICY

Price may be defined as the exchange of goods or services in terms of money. Without price there is no marketings is the society. If money is not there, exchange of goods can not be undertaken. The pricing decision of a company depends on many factors like.

(i) Marketing mix

(ii) Cost of the product

(iii) Objective/goals of the company
(iv) Demand of the product
(v) Competition
(vi) Buyers
(vii) Govt. policy

TYPES OF PRICING POLICY

(a) **Skimming pricing policy.** It involves a high introductory price in the initial stage to skim to skim the cream of demand. The products when introduced in the market have a limited period free from other manufactures. During this perioed, it aims at profit maximization according to the favourable marketing condition.

(b) **Penetration pricing policy**. A low price is designed in the initial stage with a view to capture greater market share. Because of low price the sales volume increases, competition falls down.

(c) **Zone pricing policy.** Under this, the company divides the market into zones and quotes uniform prices to all buyers who buy within a zone. The price in one zone varies from that of another zone. This is a part of geographical pricing.

FACTORS INFLUENCING PRICE

While fixing the price for his product, as entrepreneur should keep in mind the following factors:

Prices move up: Reasons

- There is more demand but less supply
- Weak competitors exist
- Factors of production are used inefficiently
- Goods are non-perishable by nature
- There is increase in wage but not in productivity
- Buyers are eager to purchase

Prices move down: Reasons

- There is more supply but less demand
- Strong competitors exist
- Factors of production are used efficiently
- Goods are perishable by nature
- Wages are stable and productivity rises
- Buyers resist purchase

CHANNELS OF DISTRIBUTION OR MARKETING CHANNEL

Definition

"A channel of distribution or marketing channel is the structure of intra-company organisation units and extra-company agents and dealers, wholesale and retail through which a company's commodity, product or service is marketed". According to American Marketing Association.

Marketing channel may also be defined as a pathway composed of intermediaries, also called middlemen, who perform such functions as needed to ensure smooth flow of goods and services from the manufacturing ends to the consuming ends in order to achieve marketing of the produce of a company.

IMPORTANCE OF CHANNEL OF DISTRIBUTION

The channel of distribution is very important to the producer and the consumer. The producer is situated at one place and the consumers are scattered in many places. The gap between the producers and consumers is shrunk by the channel of distribution.

The channel of distribution helps in making products available at the right time in the right place and in the right quantity.

TYPES OF CHANNELS OF DISTRIBUTION

1. Direct Channel of Distribution

Manufactures Consumer. In this the products are directly transferred to consumers by the manufactures. It is the shortest and simplest channel. It is adopted specifically by producers of perishable goods, or when the plant is located near the customer and it is earier to sell the products directly to them. Direct channel is also widely used wherever new products are introduced into the market for aggressive sales and for goods of technical nature which need demonstration and therefore can be marketed directly.

The following are the methods used by producer, under direct channel :

(i) Opening sales counter at manufacturing plant

(ii) Door to door sales

(iii) Sales by mail order method

(iv) Sales by opening own shops

2. Indirect Channel

In this channel middlemen or intermediaries are used between producer and consumer. It is of following types

(a) One-tier Indirect Channel

Manufacture-Retailer-Consumer

In this channel there is an intermediary retailer. A manufacturer sells goods to consumers through these retailers.

If the buyers are large, this channel is preferrable. automobile appliances, clothings, shoes etc. are sold directly to retailers.

(b) Two-tier Indirect Channel

Manufactures-Wholesalers-Retailer-Consumer

Wholesaler and retailers are the two types of intermediary in this channel. A manufacture channels his products to consumers through those intermediaries. the wholesalers are being used here because they have more finance and knowledge of marketing and selling compared to retailer only.

(c) Three-tier Indirect Channel

Manufactures-Agent/Middlemen/Wholesalers-Retailer-Consumer

In this three types of intermediaries are used. The gap between the manufactures and the consumers is very great. In this channel, the manufactures uses the services of the agent/middlemen/sales agent for the disperal of goods. The agent distributes the goods to the wholesalers who sells the goods to retailer and who in turn sells it to the consumers.

MARKETING PROBLEMS OF SSI

1. Competition from large scale section.
2. Lack of sales promotion.
3. Weak bargaining power.
4. Lack of infrastructure and finance for marketing.
5. Lack of expertise in marketing.

ADVERTISING

DEFINITION

1. It is a mass communication of information intended to persuade buyers as to maximise profits.
2. Advertising consists of all the activities in presenting to a group a non-personal, oral or visual, openly sponsored message regarding a product, service or idea.

FEATURES OF ADVERTISING

1. A message to large groups.
2. Non-personal communication (i.e., not delivered by actual person and not addressed to a single person).
3. Persuades the buyers (i.e., a type of persuasion).
4. Paid form of publicity (paid for by advertisers to publisher).

ADVERTISING MEDIA

It is a means through which the advertising message is conveyed to the consumers. proper selection of media depends on following factors :

1. Nature and type of customers (nature of segments)
2. The objectives of communication
3. Fund available for advertising
4. Characteristics of the product and its demand
5. The nature and extent of competition prevailing etc.

TYPES OF MEDIA

1. Indoor advertising (Press, Radio, TV, Handbills)
2. Outdoor advertising (Poster, Displays, Leaflets etc.)
3. Direct advertising (Sales letter, Store publications)
4. Promotional or display advertising (Window display, Exhibitions etc.)

1. Indoor advertising

When advertising is made through newspapers, magazines, radio, TV programmes etc. So that people can get the message at home is known as indoor advertising.

2. Outdoor advertising

It passes the message to those people who are moving audience. Generally, almost all the people go out on some purpose or other, e.g., office, walk, sight seeing etc. This is one of the best type of advertising as its permanent, low cost and always attracts viewers, because of its style and colourful appearance.

Types. Posters, Advertising Boards, Vehicular Advertising, Electric Display, Leaflets (Handbills) etc.

3. Direct advertising

The object of direct adverting is to create a direct contact with the customers. The advertiser can keep a close touch with the customer or the public, who are supposed to, have interest in his product through mail advertising. In this written form of communication, i.e., letters are used. Its merits are that a personal relationship with the customers can be maintained.

Types. Sales letters, Circulars, Booklets and Catalogues etc.

4. Promotional advertising

The object of promotional advertising is to increase the sales. These are also known as display advertising. In this the products are systematically kept in a place so as to attract the attention and notice of the lookers. It is beneficial as it attracts the onlooker and the whole shop looks attractive. It is flexible and consumers can study the product and its functions at leisure.

Types. Window Display, Indoor Display (glass closed upboard), Showrooms and Exhibitions etc.

OBJECTIVES OF ADVERTISING

1. To do the entire selling job (as in mail order advertising).
2. To introduce a new product (by building brand awareness among potential buyers).
3. To force middlemen to handle the product (pull strategy).

4. To build brand preference (by making it more difficult for middlemen to sell substitutes).
5. To remind users to buy the product (retentive strategy).
6. To popularise some change in marketing strategy (change in price, etc.).
7. To combat or neutralise competitor's advertising.
8. To acquaint buyers and prospects with the new uses of the product (to extend the product's life cylce).

In sum the primary objectives of advertising is to increase sales.

FUNCTIONS OF ADVERTISING

The main objective of advertising is to increase sales to all customers-present, former and future. Advertising increases the present sales and potential demand of the product. The above objectives are realised by the functions of advertising. These are

I. Increasing the Number of Customers

(a) **By increasing the customers and widening the market.** Advertising through communication media informs consumers about the presence of a product in the market. This works in two ways. First it stimulates demand and then it strengthens the stimulated demand. Thus it serves to widen the market by increasing the buyers.

(b) **By developing a brand loyalty.** All manufactures aim to attract prospects in favor of their products and services. Development of loyalty to one's brand among the customers is important. For example, if one is using a particular brand of soap, then advertising must aim at making him to use only this soap.

(c) **Offset the competing brands.** Advertising facilitates the creation, direction and extension of demand for the particular products or services. Many similar products are flowing towards the market and consumers are tempted to buy them through various promotional measures. By focusing the qualities and merits of the product in a better way than other similar products, the competitors can be defeated by capturing their share of the market.

II. Increasing the Consumption Rate Among Present Consumer

(a) **Increasing usage of the product.** Advertising helps in explaining the multiple uses of product to the masses.

(b) **Reminding the consumers.** For products like woolen dresses, air-coolers etc. which are seasonal. During season they are saleable but during off season, nil sales may be possible. At the arrival of season, customers may not remember the brand used by them before. In these circumstances, advertising reminds the customers about the forgotten products.

(c) **Educating the public.** Advertising is a link between producers and consumers. It plays a role of imparting knowledge about the good or bad reactions of certain product or services to the consumers, e.g., shampoo, hair dye, soap, baby milk powder, hair oil, medicine etc. The understanding of the product, its uses, advantage etc. can be well educated through advertising.

(d) **Shaping a goodwill.** Almost every firm wants to establish a good name in the society. The consumer may prefer a product because of its low price, fashion, after sales service, multiple uses, quality etc., All these merits are known to the consumers through advertising and sales are boosted automatically. Thus a firm can build a goodwill for its products.

Advantages of Advertising

Advertising is considered multi-dimensional. It helps is number of marketing activities. It is a technique of sales promotion. It is advantages to:

I. Advantages to Manufactures

(a) It increases the sales volumes
(b) It increases the net profit
(c) It controls product price
(d) It helps is opening new market
(e) It maintain the existing market
(f) It creates reputation
(g) It is less expensive

Manufacturers can change the habits and prejudices of customers by tactful advertising. Thus, it helps in establishing and controlling the buyer habits of the customers.

II. Advantages to Salesman

(a) Creates a background
(b) Advertised product can be sold easily
(c) Curtails the burden of the salesman's job

III. Advantages to Wholesalers and Retailers

(a) Creates easy sales (attracts more customers)
(b) Increases the turn over
(c) Publicity

IV. Advantages to Customers

(a) Easy purchasing
(b) Saves time
(c) Educates the customer

(d) Advertising is the connecting link between the manufacturer and the customers. It eliminates the middlemen.

V. Advantage to Community

(a) Increases employment opportunities

(b) Uplifts the standard of living

(c) Educative value

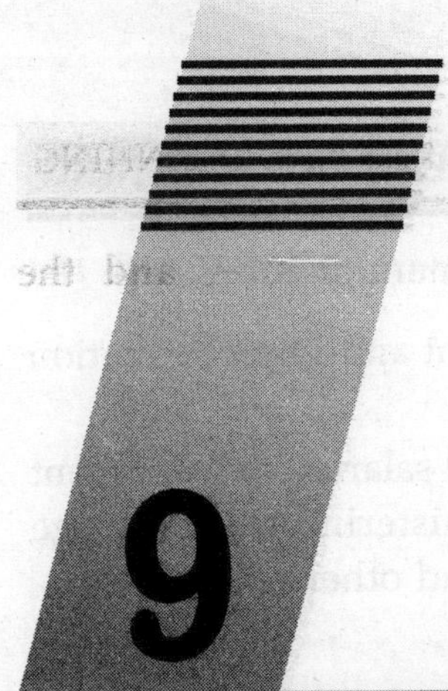

9 HUMAN RESOURCE MANAGEMENT (HRM)

Human resource management is concerned with the management of people at work.

DEFINITION

1. HRM refers to the philosophy, policies, procedures and practices related to the management of people within the organisation.
2. HRM is the planning, organising, directing and controlling of the procurement, development, compensation, integration, maintenance and separation of Human Resources to the end that individual, organisational and societal objectives are accomplished.

Aspects of HRM are

1. *Labor/personel aspect.* Concerned with recruitment, placement, remuneration, promotion, incentive etc.
2. *Welfare aspect.* Concerned with working conditions, such as canteen, creches, housing schools, recreation, housekeeping and personal problems of workers.
3. *Industrial relation aspect.* Concerned with Trade Union negotiations, settlement of I.D., and collective bargaining etc.

MAJOR ACTIVITIES UNDER HRM

1. MPP/HRP
2. Acquisition of HR (Recruitment and Selection)
3. Motivation
4. T and D (Training and development)
5. Compensation and benefits
6. Managing performance
7. Labor relations
8. Employee records

WAGE AND SALARY ADMINISTRATION

Wage and salary admininistration refers to the establishment and implementation of sound policies and practices fo employee compensation.

It includes such areas as job evaluation, surveys of wage and salaries, development and maintence of wage structure, establishing rules for administering wages, wage payment, incentives, profit sharing, supplementary payments and other related item.

Objectives:

1. The basic purpose of wage and salary administration is to establish and maintain an equitable wage and salary structure.
2. The establishment and maintance of an equitable labor cost structure, i.e., optimal balancing of conflicting personnel interests so that satisfaction of employers and employees is maximised and conflicts minimized.
3. Utilization of wages and salaries as an incentive to greater employee productivity.
4. Control of costs.

Compensation. Money received in the performance of work plus the many kinds of benefits and services that organisation provide their employees.

Wages—renumeration paid (mainly hours) for the service of labour in production etc. i.e. blue collar (workers)
Salary—weekly or monthly rates paid to clerks, administration or professional employees i.e., white collar employees.

Indirect compensation benefits, consists of life, accident and health insurance, employers contribution to retirement, pay for vaccation etc.

Wage levels. It represent the money an average worker make in a geographic area or in his organisation (it is only an average).

FACTORS INFLUENCING WAGE AND SALARY STRUCTURE AND ADMINISTRATION

A sound wage policy is to adopt a job evaluation programme in order to establish fair differentials in wages based upon differences in job contents.

Besides the basic factors provided by a job description and job evaluation, those that are usually taken into consideration for wage and salary administration are:-

1. The organisation's ability to pay
2. Supply and demand of labours
3. The prevailing market rate

4. The cost of living
5. Productivity
6. Trade Union's Bargaining Power
7. Job requirements
8. Managerial attitude

ADMINISTRATION OF WAGE AND SALARIES

To achieve the objectives of wage and salary administration the responsibility for wage and salary administration (usually) lies with the top management. The HR managers play an important role in developing the wage policies and procedures. In many organisations the task is entrusted to wage and salary committee composed of line and staff executives. The major functions of such committee are:-

(i) Approval and/or recommendation to management on job evaluation methods and findings.

(ii) Review and recommend basic wage and salary structure.

(iii) Help in formation of wage policies.

(iv) Co-ordination and review of relative departmental rates to ensure conformity/uniformity.

(v) Review of budget estimates for wage and salary adjustments and increases.

This committee should be supported by the advice of the technical staff. Such staff committees may be for job evaluation, job description, wage and salary surveys in an industry, and for a review of present wage rates, procedure and policies.

The over-all plan is first prepared by the HR managers in consultation and discussions with senior member of other departments. It is then submitted for final approval to the top executive. (Once he has given his approval, for the wage and salary structure and the rules for administration, its implementation becomes a joint effort of all heads of the department.)

PRINCIPLES OF WAGE AND SALARY ADMINISTRATION

The generally accepted principles governing the function of wages and salary are:

1. Wage policies should be carefully developed, having in mind the interests of management (as representatives of owners) the employees, the consumers and the community.
2. Wage policies should be clearly expressed in writing to ensure uniformity and stability.
3. Wage decisions should be checked against the carefully formulated policies.
4. Management should see to it that the employees know and understand the wage policies.

5. Wage policies should be evaluated from time to make certain that they are adequate for current needs.
6. Departmental performance should be checked periodically against the standards set in advance.
7. Job descriptions and performance ratings should be checked periodically to keep them update.

METHODS OF WAGE PAYMENT AND INCENTIVE PLAN

Their are two principal systems of wage payments:

(a) **Time wage system.** Under this system, the workers is paid for the amount of time spent on the job. This is the oldest and most common system and the wages are based on a certain period of time during the course of work. The period of time may be an hour, a day, a week, a fornight, or a month and the wage rate will depend upon the period of time. Wages are paid after the time fixed for work is completed, irrespective of output or completion of the work.

So, Wages = No. of hours worked × Rate per hour.

Advantages:

1. **Simplicity.** It is simple, for the amount earned by a worker can be easily calculated.
2. **Quality of work.** As their is no time limit for the execution of a job, workmen are not in a hurry to finish it and this mean that they will pay attention to their work.
3. **Equality.** As all the workmen employed for doing a particular kind of work receive the same wages, illfeeling and jealousy among them are avoided.
4. **Less wastage/rough use of machines.** Due to slow and steady pace of the worker, there is no rough handling of machines, which is advantageous for the employer.
5. **Feeling of security.** It gives the worker a feeling of security as he knows in advance what will be his total pay at the end of the period.
6. This is the only system that can be used profitably where the output of an individual workman or groups of employee cannot be readily measured.

Disadvantages:

1. **Lack of motivation.** This system doesnot take into account the fact that men are of different abilities and if all workmen are paid equally, better workmen will have no incentive to work harder and better.
2. This system does not check employeer inefficiency as there is no link between wages and productivity.

3. **Need for close supervision.** Time wage system leads to lower productivity unlesss strict supervision is provided. Thus, there is a need of close supervision to ensure better productivity.

(b) **Piece-wage system.** In this system output of work is the basis of wage payment. A worker is paid according to the amount of work completed or the number of units turned out irrespective of the time taken. (Though the time is not essence, here it is assumed that the worker will not take more than average time to complete the job.)

So, Wages = No. of units produced × Rate per unit.

The rate per unit remains the same irrespective of the number of units produced. It is then called as straight piece rate system.

F.W. Taylor (1906) introduced differential Piece Rate System. In this two different wages are prescribed – higher and lower. The highes piece rate is meant for efficient worker and the lower for inefficient workers who produce less than the standard quota.

Merits:

1. Incentive for higher production

This system privides incentive to better workers to produce more (It pays workman according to his efficiency).

2. Costing

Costing of production becomes easier as wages are a constant factor for each unit of production or as the direct labor cost per unit of production becomes easy, calculation of cost become easy.

Wage Incentives

1. The term wage incentives refers to objective in the internal situation whose function is to increase or maintain, some already initiated activity, either in duration or in intensity.
2. It refer to all the plans that provides extra pay for extra performance in addition to regular wages for a job.

A wage incentive scheme is essentially a managerial device of increasing a worker's productivity. Incentive wages relate earnings to productivity. It may use premium, bonus or a variety of rates to compensate for superior performance.

Objectives of Wage Incentive Schemes

1. To improve the profit of a firm through reduction in the unit costs of labor or material or both.
2. To avoid or minimize additional capital investment for the expansion of production capacity.

3. To increase a workers earnings without dragging the firm into a higher wage rate structure regardless of productivity.
4. To use wage incentives as a useful tool for securing a better utilization of manpower, better production scheduling and performance control.

KINDS OF INCENTIVE PLANS

Broadly the various incentive plans can be classified into two plans:

(A) Individual Incentive Plans

(B) Group Incentive Plans

A. Individual Incentive Plans

Time based. Under time based incentive plans, a standard time is determined for doing a job. A standard time serves as the basis for giving bonus to the worker if they meet or exceed the standard. A worker is said to be efficient if he completes his job in less than standard time. In order to reward him for his efficiency he may given bonus under an appropriate incentive plan. For example, Halsey plan, Rowan plan etc.

1. Halsey Plan

Halsey premium plan is simple combination of time and speed basis of payment. Under this plan, a minimum time wage is guaranteed to every worker. A limited time is fixed for the completion of a job. If a worker performs his job in less than standard time, he is given bonus. But there is no penalty for performing the job in more than the standard time fixed. The slow worker is paid the time wages and the efficient worker is paid some bonus in additional to the time wage. (The bonus is in proportion of the wages which he could have earned during the time saved.)

For example, standard time (S) = 12 hrs

Time taken by a worker (T) = 8 hours

Rate of wages (R) = 9 Rs. per hour

Bonus (P) = Wages for 50% of the time saved

Total wages (W) = S × R + 50% of (S – T) × R

$$= 8 \times 9 + \frac{50}{100} \times 4 \times 9$$

= Rs. 90

2. Rowan Plan

The Rowan plan is a modification of the Halsay plan. It also guarantees the minimum time wages and does not penalise a slow worker. A standard time is fixed for completion of a job and bonus is paid to a worker on the bais of time saved. Here, the bonus is that proportion of the wages for the time taken which the time saved bears to the standards time.

Efficiency is thus measured as $= \frac{\text{Time Saved}}{\text{Std. time}}$

As the time saved increases, time taken will be reduced and as such the bonus would increase at a diminishing rate. This will check over-speeding and overcome the major drawback of Halsay plan.

Standard time (S) = 12 hours

Time taken by a worker (T) = 8 hours

Rate of wages (R) = Rs. 9 per hour

Total wages $(W) = S \times R + \left(R \times \frac{\text{Time Save}}{\text{Std. time}}\right)$

$= 11 \times 9 + \left(9 \times \frac{4}{12}\right)$

$= 08 + 3 = 111$

(ii) **Production based incentive plans.** In this a standard of output is determined on scientific basis and payment of wages is made on the basis of number of units produced by a worker. A higher rate per unit is paid to the efficient worker.

Production based incentive plans include.

1. Taylor's Differential Piece Rate System

In this plan Taylor suggested two piece rates for the workers. The lowes rate for those who give production below the standard workload and higher piece rate for those who give production above the standard workload fixed.

For example

Standard units to produce = 40

For 40 units and above = 1 Re.

For less than 40 units = 90 paise

2. Merrick's Multiple Piece Rate Plan

This plan offer three grade piece rates rather than two offered by Taylor's plan.

(i) The workers who produce less than 83% of standard output are paid at a basic piece rate.

(ii) Those producing from 83% to 100% of the standard output are paid 110% of basic piece rate.

(iii) Workers producing more than 100% of standard output are paid 120% of basic piece rate.

For example

Standard output = 100 units

Piece rate = 10 paise

Case (i)

Output = 80 units

$$\text{Efficiency} = \frac{80}{100} \times 100 = 80\%$$

So, wages = 80×0.10

(as less than 83%) = Rs. 8.00

Case (ii)

Output = 90 units

$$\text{Efficiency} = \frac{90}{100} \times 100 = 90\%$$

$$\text{Earnings} = 90 \times \frac{100}{100} \times 0.10$$

(more than 83%) = Rs. 9.90

Case (iii)

Output = 110 units

$$\text{Eff.} = \frac{110}{100} \times 100 = 110\%$$

So earnings

$$= 110 \times \frac{120}{100} \times 0.10$$

= Rs. 13.20

GROUP INCENTIVE PLANS

A fundamental assumption common to all individual schemes is that the output of each worker can be accurately measured. But in some cases, for example in the grinding and welding works in the electrical industry, the operations are performed by the groups. As a whole, and the contribution of each worker in the group cannot be accurately, measured. In such cases, the groups incentive schemes are followed. For example :

1. Profit Sharing Method

The total earnings of a group are first determined in accordance with the incentive method which is followed (any of the individual incentive plan), and the earnings are then distributed among the members of the groups on some equitable basis. If the groups consists of member with equal skills, the earnings are divided equally among them. When the member are of unequal skill, the earnings of group may be divided among the member in proportion to their individual time rates or according to specified percentage.

Pre-requisites of a good wage incentive plan. There are several conditions necessary for successful implementation of incentive wage plan. These are:

1. **Suitable climate** i.e., good relations between management and labours.
2. **Clear and complete information to goals,** i.e., clear objectives and clear rate and caluculation of bonus.
3. **Simplicity.** The plan introduced must be simple and easy for worker to calculate and to understand.
4. **Inexpressive.** Scheme should not involve maintence of elaborate records etc.
5. **Just and equitable.** Wage system should be just and equitable to both employee and employer.

6. **Scientifically set standards.** The norms on which plans is based should be fixed through careful and scientific approach.
7. **Elasticity.** Scheme should have elasticity to take care of technical and other changes as to rectify error.
8. **Stability.** standards and rates once fixed should not be frequently changed unless substantial change.
9. **Ensure** that effort and rewards are directly related.

2. Employee Stock Ownership Plan (ESOP)

Under the most basic form of employee stock ownership plan (ESOP) a corporation contributes shares of its own stock, or cash to be used to purchase such stock to a trust, established to purchase shares of the firm's stock for employees.

These centributions are generally made annually in proportion to total employee compensation, with a limit of 15% of compensation.

The trust holds the stock in individual employee accounts and distributes it to employee upon retirement or other separation from service (assuming the employee has worked long enough to earn ownership of the stock).

Advantage. The corporation receive a tax deduction equal to the share market value of the shares that are transferred to the trustee. Employees are not taxed until they receive a distribution from the trust, usually at retirement when their tax rate is reduced.

ESOP's encourage employees to develop a sense of ownership in and commitment to the firm.

NON-FINANCIAL INCENTIVES

It is a well established fact now that an individual doesnot work for money alone. He requires certain non-financial incentive also which satisfy his social, psychological and personal growth needs.

Some of them are (individual) :

1. Status
2. Promotion
3. Responsibility and challenge
4. Recognition of work
5. Job security

GROUP

1. Social importance of work
2. Team spirit
3. Healthy competition

4. Informal group (informal relations)
5. Leadership

Council. Money is not the only motivator. The employees being human beings are mored to act become of certain non-rational factors also. They respond to their environment, in term of such factors as hopes and fears, like and dislikes, irritation, success etc. They need non-financial incentives to satisfy their socio-psychological needs and their personal growth and development needs.

People need not only the "skill to work" but also the "will to work" which comes through incentive both financial as well as non-financial.

EMPLOYEE BENEFITS

Financial incentives are paid to specific employees whose work is above standard "Employee benefits are available to all employees based on their membership in the organisation".

The purpose of such benefits is to retain people in the organisation. These foster loyalty and act as a security base for the worker.

DEFINITION

Fringe benefit is primarily a means in the direction of ensuring, maintaing and increasing the income of the employee. It is a benefit which supplements to a worker's ordinary wages (and which is of value to them and their families in so far as it materially increases there retirement).

Wages	Fringe Benefits
1. Wages are directly related to work done and are paid regularly usually weekly or monthly.	1. Fringe benefit are those payments or benefits which a worker enjoys in addition to the wages or salary he received.
2. These are paid to the workers for the specific job they have performed.	2. These benefits are not given to worker for any specific jobs they have performed but are offered to them to stimulate there interest in work.
3. These are not extra cost to the employer as they are directly related to work done.	3. Fringe benefit represents a labours cost for the employee, for it is an expenditure which he incurs on supplementing the average money rates due to his employees.

4. It is a direct reward for the output. It is offered on the basis of the hard work or long hours of work put in by an employee.	4. It is never a direct reward geared to the output, effort or merit of an employee. But it is on the basis of length of service, his sickness the hazards of life he encountered in the course of his work etc.

If the benefit increases a worker's efficiency, it is not a fringe, but if it is given to supplement his wages, it is a fringe benefit.

For example, the expenditure's incurred on providing better lighting arrangements with a view to increase a worker's efficiency is not counted as expendicture on fringe even though workers may gain financially as a result of this increased efficiency because of better lights. Subsidised meals, however constitute a fringe benefit.

Benefits. Apply to those for which items direct monetary value to the individual employee can be ascertained, e.g., pension.

Services. Such items as a company newspaper etc. for which a direct money value for the individual employee cannot be readity established.

FRINGE BENEFITS SATISFY THREE GOALS

1. Social Goal

Fringe benefits act as a social lever in helping conservation of human resource, by guarding against its unnatural erossion and providing the climate for its development in a working environment.

2. Human Relations Goal

The management, through, motivation tries to develop and maintain human relations. The management provides with an environment which will reasonably meet the economic, social and psychological needs of the employees so that there co-operation could be obtained and productivity of the organisaiton enhanced.

3. Macro-Economics Goal

For maintaining the growth and stability in the economy of a country, ideal utilization of the non-human and human resource is imperative. Fringe benefits do provide protection, during periods of contingencies of life, for T and D of employee, and for good working conditions and assistance to supplement their main income etc.

Main purpose or objective of employee benefits and services are

1. To recruit and retain the best personnel.
2. To provide for the needs of the employee and protect them against certain hazards of life (particularly those which as individual cannot himself provide for).

3. To increase and improve an employee's morale and create a helpful and positive attitude on the part of workers towards their employers.
4. To promote employee loyalty to the organisation.
5. To promote employment stabilization and employee identification with organisation.
6. To furnish and improve the organisational image in the eyes of the public with a view to improving its market position.

Employee Benefits may be classified as follows :

A. Employee security payment

(i) Employee's contribution stipulated in legal acts: old age, servivor, disability, health and unemployment insurance.

(ii) Payments under the Workman's Compensation Act.

(iii) Accident insurance

(iv) Pensions

(v) Contributions to saving plans and health and welfare funds.

B. Payment for time not worked

Under these are included clear up time, health is the family, leave, holiday pay off, lay off pay, medical time, paid lunch period, pay for religious holidays, pay for rest periods, severance pay (i.e., money given after termination), paid sick leave, payment for time spent on collecting bargaining, vacation pay etc.

C. Bonus and awards

Includes such financial amenities and advantages as holiday, overtime, Diwali bonus (bonus for good quality workmanship), safety awards, suggestion awards, and year end bonus.

EMPLOYEE SERVICES

In addition to the employee benefits, employee services are also provided by the organisation at no cost to the employee or at a significant reduction from what he might have to pay without the organisation support. Following are four broad types of employee services.

1. Professional

Professional services are offered to employee in various aspects like legal aid, vocational guidance, employee counselling etc.

2. Recreational and social services

Recreation and social services include social get-togethers, informal association, duties, sports, picnics, cultural activities, libraries, reading rooms etc.

3. Employee conveniences

(Some of there are required by law whereas some are demanded by the unions) There include canteens (according to Factories Act 1948, for more then 250 employees) housing services (i.e., company owned housing projects and subsidized housing), transportation services, purchasing services (i.e., discount on company products and services), medical services (i.e., clinics, hospitals etc.); educational services indude sponsorship for off-duty course, tuition fee refunds, scholarships for employees and their children.

4. Auxiliary services

These are other miscellaneous service gifts. Employee are given gifts on certain occasions like Diwali, Community Service Activities (Blood Donation, Programmes, Famine or Drought Relief Fund and other charity services), Employee Publication (including house journals, pamphlets and bulletins containing information on severals matters of interest to employees); Loan Services (for illness, accident any financial emergency, marriage, child birth, house repair etc.).

Disadvantages:

1. **Expensive.** Also may are not always lie the benefits that want. Under most conditions the individual employee is forced to take the whole fringe packet whether or not it meets his individual needs.
2. **Continued demand for additional benefits.** Employees start demanding them as their right, which is not really so.
3. Many a time in its desire to let employees know what the organisation is doing for their welfare, management may create the impression of being paternalistic. So employees then do not receive these benefits with full enthusiasm.
4. **Maintence of the least productive worker.** With an increase in benefits and services, employees, particularly when they are not very productive tend to stick to their jobs (and are not interested in changing them).

PERFORMANCE APPRAISAL

DEFINITION

Performance appraisal is evaluation or measurement of performance against some defined jobs.

APPRAISING WORK EFFECTIVENESS

The system's appraisal and record practices influence attitude and behavior of employees in organisation.

PURPOSE OF PERFORMANCE APPRAISAL

Performance appraisal serves a number of purposes in organisation. These are:

1. Appraisals provide information for such important decisions as promotions, transfer and terminations.
2. Appraisals identify T and D needs. They pinpoint employee skills and competencies that are currently inadequate but can be remedied if appropriate programmes are developed.
3. Performance appraisals can be used as a criterion against which selection and development programmes are validated. (Newly hired employees who perform poorly can be identified through performance appraisal.)
4. Appraisals also fulfill the purpose of providing feedback to employees on how the organisation views their performance.
5. Finally, performance appraisals are used as the basis for reward allocations. Decisions about who gets merit pay increases and other rewards are typically determined by performance appraisals.

PERFORMANCE APPRAISAL AND MOTIVATION

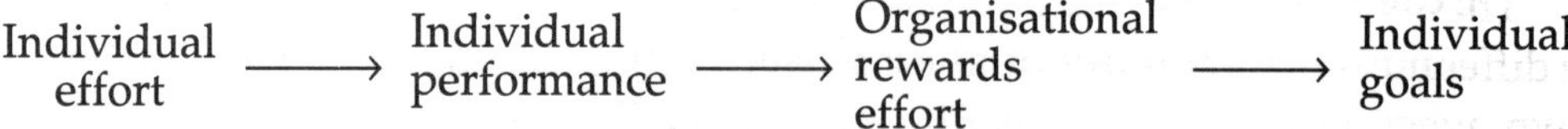

The strength of a person's motivation to perform (effort) depends on how strongly he believes that he can achieve what he attempts. If he achieves his goals (performance), will he be adequately rewarded and, if he is rewarded by the organisattion will the reward satisfy his individual goals ?

The above model (expectancy theory of motivation) offers the best explanation of what conditions the amount of effort an individual will exert on his or her job. A vital component of this model is performance, specifically the effort performance and performance reward linkages. Do people see effort as leading to performance, and performance to the rewards that they value. Clearly, (1) they have to know what is expected of them. (2) They need to know how their performance will be measured. Further, they must feel (3) confident that if they exert an effort within their capabilities, it will result in a satisfactory performance as defined by the criteria by which they are being measured. Finally, (4) They must feel confident that if they perform as they are being asked, they will achieve the rewards they value.

In brief, if the objectives that employees are seeking are unclear, if the criteria for measuring those objectives are vague, and if the employees lack confidence that their efforts will lead to a satisfactory appraisal of this appraisal, or believe there will be an unsatisfactory pay off by the organisation when this performance objectives are achieved, we can enpect individual to work considerable below their potential.

OBJECTIVE OF P.A

- Allocate resources
- Motivate and reward employees
- Give employee feedback
- Maintain fairness
- Coach and develop employees
- Comply with equal employment opportunity regulations.

METHODS OF P.A

1. Written essays

The simplest method of appraisal is to write a narrative describing an employee's strengths, weaknesses, past performance, potential and suggestions for improvement (so good or bad appraisal may be determined as much by the evaluation's writing skill as by the employee's actual level of performance).

2. Critical incidents

These focus on the evaluator's attention on those behaviours that are key in making the difference between executings a job effectively or ineffectively, i.e., the appraiser writes down anecdotes that describe what the employee did that was specifically effective or ineffective. The key here is that only specific behaviors, and not vaguely defined personality traits, are cited.

3. Graphic rating scales

This is one of the oldest and most popular methods. In this method, a set of performance factors, such as quality and quantity of work, depth of knowledge, co-operation, loyalty, attendance, honesty and initiative are tested. The evaluator then goes down the list and rates each on incremental scales. The scales typically specify five points, so a factor such as job knowledge might be rated 1 (''poorly informed about work duties'') to 5 (''has complete mastery of all phases of the job'').

This method is popular because it is less time consuming and allows for quantitative analysis and comparison.

4. Multiperson comparison

These evaluate one individual's performance against that of one or more others. It is a relative rather than absolute measuring device. The three most popular comparisons are group order ranking, individual ranking and paired comparisons.

The group order ranking require the evaluator to place employees into a particular classification, such as top one-fifth or second one-fifth and so on. This method is often used in recommending students to graduate schools or campus interviews.

The individual ranking approach rank orders employees from best to worst. If the manager is required to appraise thirty, subordinates, this approach assumes that the difference between the first and second employee is the same as that between the 21st and 22nd. The result is a clear ordering of employees, from the highest performer down to the lowest.

The paired comparisions approach compares each employee with every other employee and rates each as either the superior or the weaker member of the pair. After all paired comparions are made, each employee is assigned a summary ranking based on the number of superior scores he or she achieved.

POTENTIAL PROBLEMS

Although organisation may seek to make the performance appraisal process free from personal biases, prejudices can creep into the process for example:

1. Single criterion

The typical employee's job is made up of a number of tasks. when employees are appraised on a single job criterion, even though successful performance on that job requires good performance on several criteria, employees will concentrate on the single criterion to the enclusion of other relevant factors.

2. Leniency error

Every appraiser has his or her own value system that acts as a standard against which appraisals are made relative to the true or actual performance of an individual. Some evaluators mark high and other low. The former is referred to as positive leniency error and the latter as negative leniency error. (In positive leniency the performance is overstated and vice versa).

If all individuals in an organisation were appraised by the same person, there would be no problem. Although there would be an error factor, it would be applied equally to everyone. The difficulty arises when we have different raters with different leniency errors making judgements.

3. Halo error

This is the tendency for an evaluator to let the assessment of an individual on one trait influence his or her appraisal of that person on other traits For example, if an employee tends to be trustworthy and dependable, we might become biased toward that individual and rate him high on many other desirable attributes.

4. Similarity error

When evaluators rate other people by giving special consideration to those qualities that they perceive in themselves, they are making a similarity error. For example evaluators who see themselves as aggressive may appraise other by looking for aggressiveness.

GRIEVANCES

DEFINITION

Grievances means any discontent or dissatisfaction, whether expressed or not and whether valid or not, arising out of anything connected will the company that an employee thinks, believes or even feels, is unfair, unjust or inequitable.

CAUSES

1. Economic

Wage fixation, wage calculation, overtime, bonus etc. Employees feel that they are getting less than they ought so get.

2. Work environment

Poor working condition, defective equipment, machines, tools, materials etc.

3. Supervision

Boss's attitude, favouration, biasing etc.

4. Work groups

Strained relations or incompatibility with colleages feeling of neglect, victimization etc.

5. Work organisation

Rigid and unfair rules, too much or too less responsibility, lack of work appreciation/ recognition etc.

EFFECTS OF GRIEVANCES

On Prodution

- Low quality of production
- Income is wastages
- Spoilage

On Employees

- Increase rate of absenteeism and turn over
- Increase in accidents
- Decrease in employee morale

On Management

- Strained superior subordinates relation
- Increase in indiscipline cases
- Increase in unrest

DISCOVERY OF GRIEVANCES

Grievances can be uncovered in a number of ways. Gossip and grapesine offer vital clues about employee grievances. Various methods of discovering grievances are:

(a) **Observation.** A manager can usually track the behavior of people working under him (any change in behaviour is the indication).

(b) **Gripe boxes/complaint boxes.** Complant boxes may be kept at prominent positions in the factory for lodging aronymous complaints pertaining to any aspect relating to work.

(c) Exit interviews.

(d) **Open door policy.** This is a kind of walk in meeting with the seniors when the employee can express his feelings openly about any work related grievance.

(e) **Opinion surveys.** Surveys may be conducted periodically to elicit the opinions of employees about the organisation and its policies.

(f) **Grievance procedure.** A systematic grievance procedure is the best means to highlight employee dissatisfaction at various levels.

STEPS IN GRIEVANCE PROCEDURE

(i) **Identify grievances.** Employee dissatisfaction should be identified by the managers if they are not expressed.

(ii) **Define correctly.** Management ha sto define the problem properly and accurately, after it is identified/acknowledged.

(iii) **Collect data.** Complete information should be collected from all the parties relating to the grievance. Information should be classified as facts, data, opinions etc.

(iv) **Analyse and solve.** Information should be analysed, alternative standard to the problem should be developed and best solution selected.

(v) **Prompt redressal.** The grievance should be redressed by implementing the solution.

(iv) **Follow up.** Implementation and follow-up of the solution must be followed up at every stage in ordes to ensure effective and speedy implementation.

GREIVANCE REDRESSAL PROCEDURE

It is very important to settle grievances

(i) Promptly

(ii) As near as possible to the point of origin

(iii) On merit only

(iv) With as many facts as possible

(v) With as attitude of mutual confidence and respect. Hence it is useful to adopt a systematic mehod for grievance redressal.

A systematic grievance redressal producre must have the following features :

(i) It should be simple, fair and easy to understand.

(ii) It should be in writing.

(iii) It should specify to whom employees may take a grievance in the first instance.

(iv) It should state where, in the event of the grievance remaining unresolved, an employee should then address his complaint.

(v) It should specify time limits within which the aggrieved employee can expect to be noticied of the outcome of his complaint.

(vi) It should have regular meetings of the grievance committee and a record of proceedings properly minuted should be sent to all the parties.

(vii) It should promote healthy relations between employee and the company.

Model Grievance Redressal Procedure

Generally organisation have following grievance redresial procedure called as STEP LADDER Procedure.

Under this procedure, the aggrieved employee has to proceed step by step in getting his grievances heard and redressed.

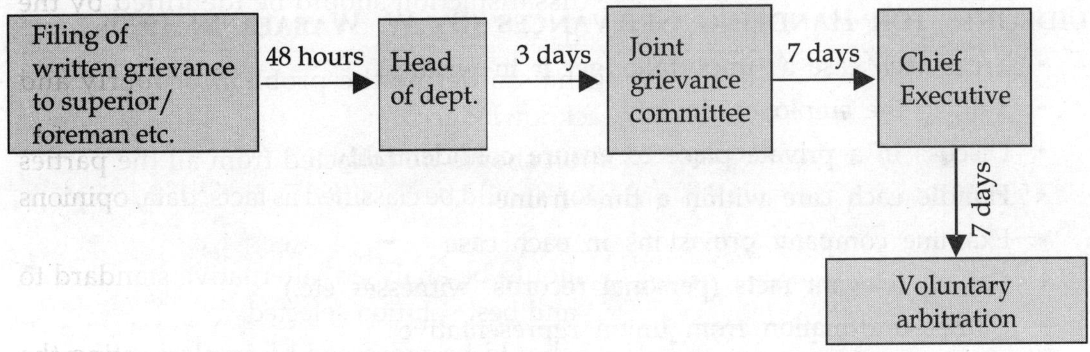

Fig. Steps in Model Grievance Redressal Procedure (with time span).

ESSENTIALS OF A GOOD GRIEVANCE PROCEDURE

1. A grievance should be dealt with in the first instance at the lowest level, i.e., with, the immediate superior.
2. It must be made clear to the employee what line of appeal is, so that if he cannot get satisfaction from his immediate superior, he may know the next higher authority to whom he can go.
3. Grievances should be dealt speedily because delay causes frustration and tempers may rise and rumors may spread around the work.
4. The grievance procedure should be set up with the participation of the employees and it should be applicable to all in the organisation.

GRIEVANCE MANAGEMENT IN INDIA (IN SSI)

At present there are three legislations dealing with grievances of employees working in industries

1. **The Industrial Employment (Standing orders) Act, 1946** requires that every organisation employing 100 or more worker should frame standing orders. These should contain, among other things, a provision for nedressal of grievances of workers against unfair treatment and wrongful actions by the employers or his agents.
2. **The Factories Act, 1948** provides for the appointment of a welfare officer in every factory employing 500 or more workers. These welfare officers also look after complaints and grievances of workers.
3. **The Industrial Disputes Act, 1947** (amended in 1965) deal with discharge, dismissal or retrenchment of employees.

In India, a Model Grievance Procedure was adopted by the Indian Labour Conference (ILC) in its 16th session held in 1958. At present, Indian companies are adopting either the Model Grievance Procedure or procedures formulated by themselves with modification in it. (This grievance procedures are mostly voluntary.)

GUIDELINES FOR HANDLING GRIEVANCES (BY W. WABAER IN 1970)

- Treat each case as important (get it in writing)
- Talk to the employee directly
- Discuss in a private place to ensure confidentiality
- Handle each care within a time frame
- Examine company provisions in each case
- Get all relevant facts (personal records, witnesses etc.)
- Gather information from union representatives
- Control your emotions, remarks and behaviour
- Maintain proper records and follow up action.

INDUSTRIAL RELATIONS

DEFINITION

1. It is that part of management which is concerned with the manpower of the organisation.
2. The fields of IR includes the study of workers and their trade unions, management, employee's associations and the state institutions concerned with the regulation of employment.

PARTIES TO INDUSTRIAL RELATIONS

1. Workers and their organisation

The personal characteristics of workers, their culture, educational attainments, qualification skills, attitude, towards work etc. play an important role in IR. Also the worker's organisations known as Trade Unions put pressure on the management for safeguarding the interests of the workers.

2. Employers and their organisation

The employers provide employment to workers and try to regulate their behavior for getting high productivity from them. Industrial unrest generally arises when the employer's demands from the workers are very high and they offer low economic and other benefits to the workers. In order to increases their bargaining powers, employee in several industries have organised employer's association. These associations put pressure on TU's and the Govt.

3. Government

The government or state exerts an important influence on IR through such measures as providing employment, interviewing in working relationships and regulating wages, bonus and working conditions through various laws relating to labor. The government keeps an eye on both the TU and employer's organisation to regulate their behaviors in the interest of the nation.

INDUSTRIAL RELATIONS

In an organisation there is always the possibilities of conflicts between management and workers on various matters which destroy industrial relation. If industrial relation is not maintained perfectly, it may lead to low production and productivity, creation of tense situation, lower industrial development, loss of industrial peace and harmony etc.

Major causes of industrial disputes are:

(a) **Economic causes.** Related to more wages, D.A. bonus, better service conditions etc.

(b) **Non-economic causes.** These are further classified as

(i) **Physical causes**. Like better working conditions, supply of essential materials.

(ii) **Psychological causes**. Like unlawful lay-off and retrenchment, misbehaviour of managers to workers, defective transfer and promotions.

(iii) **Organisational causes.** Like non-recognition of unions.

MACHINERY FOR SETTLEMENT OF DISPUTES

Whenever any dispute arises between the management and the labor steps should be taken to resolve it as early as possible. The best way in the voluntary settlement of disputes. But apart for them certain legal machinery for settlement of disputes is also available.

VOLUNTARY METHODS

(1) **Collective bargaining.** It is the easiest way of settlement of industrial dispute between employer and employees without third party interference. Under this method, the representatives of both employer and employee meet together and try to settle the dispute through peaceful negotiations.

(2) **Code of discipline.** In 1958, a labor conference was held (attached by many industrialists, Government agencies, lawyers, trade unions etc.) in which a code of discipline was prepared. The code of discipline constitutes a number of guidelines for maintainence of peace and harmony in industries and prevent occurrence of disputes. The code of disciplines include:

   (a) No strike or lockout should take place without prior notice.

   (b) There should not be any damage or loss to any industrial property.

   (c) There should be education of management and workers about their obligation to each other.

   (d) These should not be any 'go slow' by the workers.

   (e) Settlement of disputes should be done an early as possible without spoiling time.

(3) **Voluntary arbitration.** Under this method both the employer and employee agree to appoint an independent third party/person as an arbitrator, who has to go into the depth of the dispute and decide the matter himself. They enter into an agreement to abide by the decision of the arbitrator, before the arbitration starts. Whenever the award of the arbitrator is made compulsory and binding on both the parties, it is known as "compulsory arbitration".

(4) **Tripartite bodies.** These are the bodies set up constituting representatives of employers, employees and Government who play a major role in the settlement of disputes between employer and employee. Such bodies put maximum emphasis on voluntary agreement on various labor problem, e.g., the Indian Labor Conference, the Standing Labor Committee, State Labor Advisory Board etc.

LEGAL MACHINERY

The Industrial Disputes Act 1947 has a lot of provisions for creation of many authorities for prevention and settlement of industrial disputes having legal power with then. These are:

(1) **Works committee.** It is usually formed in industries where one hundred or more workers are employed. This committee consists of representatives of both

the employer and the employees. This committee attempts to remove the cause of labor management conflicts and disputes through peaceful negotiations at the work level. If it is not possible to settle a dispute at the factory level by the works commitee, the dispute is referred to the conciliation officer.

(2) **Conciliation officer.** A conciliation officer is appointed to settle the dispute arising between employer and employees when the dispute is beyond the reach of works commitee. The conciliation officer has to examine all the problems relating to the disputes and submit a report to the government within 14 days. If the dispute is not settled by him, the dispute is referred to the Board of Conciliation. At the state level, labor commissioner or additional labor commissioner are appointed as conciliation officers.

(3) **Board of conciliation.** If the conciliation officer fails to resolve the dispute, the dispute is referred to the Board of Conciliation. The Government form a board consisting of equal number of representative from the employees and the employer. A chairman is appointed by the Government, who is an outsides and an independent person with adequate experience on this matter. The board has to find the possible solution to the industrial dispute. It has to submit its report to the government within two months from the date of referring the dispute to the board.

(4) **Court of enquiry**. When a particular industrial dispute could not be solved by the Board Conciliation, the Government, may appoint a Court of Enquiry to inquire into the causes of dispute and submit a report to the Government within six months. The court collects reports and witness and goes into various aspects of the dispute and find out the causes of the dispute but does nothing for the settlement of the dispute. The persons appointed by Government as Court of Enquiry are usually of the rank of High Court Judge.

(5) **Labor court**. A labor court is the final phase for the settlement of industrial disputes. It is constituted at the national level. When as industrial dispute cannot be settled by any other method mentioned above, it is referred to the labor court. It is also called as compulsory arbitration or compulsory adjudication. The award of the court should be published by the government within 30 days of the receipt of such award.

(6) **Industrial tribunal**. It is constituted by appropriate State or Central Government to deal with the problems of industrial disputes relating to wages, bonus, allowances, hours of work, profit sharing, provident fund etc. Only the justice of high courts can be appointed by the government as the chairman of industrial tribunals.

(7) **National tribunal**. Only the Central Government has the power to refer any industrial dispute to the national tribunal. Industrial disputes of national level/ importance are usually referred to the national tribunal. The decision of national tribunal is compulsory and binding on all the parties involved.

FINANCE MANAGEMENT

FINANCE FOR SMALL SCALE INDUSTRIES

Finance is said to be the lifeblood of an industry. It is needed to assemble the inputs and run the organization. Financing of small business has its unique features some of which are:

(i) **High proportion of working funds.** Due to labor intensive technology, a large proportion of total funds are required in the form of liquid assets.

(ii) **Low credit standing.** The credit worthiness of a new SSI and his owner is generally low.

(iii) **Poor documentation.** A small scale entrepreneur is rarely familiar with legal formalities involved in financing the business. He cannot afford legal experts. He therefore prefers few formalities.

(iv) **Limited personal funds.** The owners of small scale unit generally has limited personal funds. He has to therefore depend to a large extent on borrowed funds.

The various sources of finance may be broadly classified as

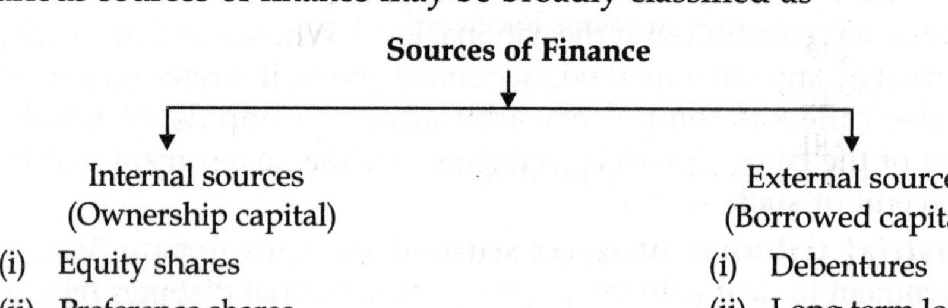

A Small Scale Industry Requires Two Types of Finance

(a) **Long term finance.** This is needed to buy fixed assets and to maintain working capital owner's capital and deposits, term loans from bank and financial institution, margin money and subsidy from Government are the sources of long term finance.

(b) **Short term finance.** Money required to meet day-to-day expenses in the scale of operations is called short term finance. Trade creditors commercial banks, customer advance and deposits from friends and relatives are the main source of short term finance.

In order to maintain the financial health of the unit, long term finance should be utilised for acquiring fixed assets and short term finance should be used for acquiring current assets.

The amount of fixed capital needed for an enterprise depends upon the following factors:

(a) Nature of business.

(b) Scale of operations or size of the enterprise.

(c) Type of manufacturing process.

(d) Cost of developing business.

(e) Technique of production.

(f) Banking facilities.

Concept of Working Capital

Working capital means the amount of funds required by an enterprise to finance its day-to-day operations. It is that part of the total capital which is employed in short term assets such as raw materials, account receivable inventory etc.

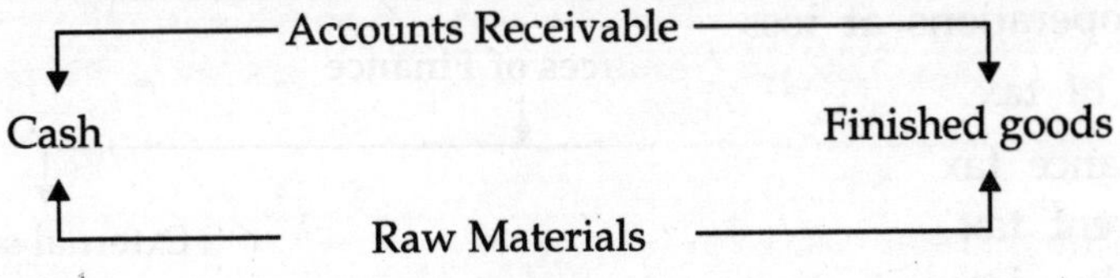

Working Capital Cycle

Working capital is required to bridge the time gap between production of goods and receipt of cash through sales. This time gap is called operating cycle of the business. During the operating cycle, working capital keeps on circulating or revolving from one form to another. Working capital is also known as 'circulating capital' or rending capital.

$$\text{Amount of working capital need} = \frac{\text{Total operating expenses in the year}}{\text{No. of operating cycles in the year}}$$

This is one of the method to estimate working capital requirements. This method is called as operating cycle method.

FUNDS FLOW ANALYSIS

Funds flow analysis help in understanding the level of working capital and its movement. Every increase or decrease of working capital is caused by funds movement from sources and applications thereof. Funds flow analysis helps to identify the various sources and application. This is helps to reveal how additional funds are created or how funds have been released. Indiscriminate release of funds for investments in fixed assets or outside business may affect normal functioning. On the other hand, unnecessary increase of funds may cause idle funds. Both increase and decrease should be supported by proper funds requirement analysis.

Funds flow analysis is made on the basis of annual profit and loss account and balance sheets as on year end dates. Funds decrease if funds inflows between two dates are less than funds outflows. To the contrary, funds will increase if the funds inflows between two dates are more than funds outflows.

Various sources of funds are:

- Issue of shares at premium/discount.
- Raising of loans.
- Sales of fixed assets; sale of investments.
- Trading operations at profit.

Various application of funds are:

- Redemption of preference shares
- Repayment of loans
- Purchase of fixed assets and investments
- Trading operations at loss
- Payment of tax
  - — Advance tax
  - — Current tax
  - — Penalty, interest etc.
- Payment of dividend.

FUNDS FLOW STATEMENT

This is a statement which shows various courses and applications together and explain reasons for changes in working capital (non-cash adjustments of liabilities and assets do not involve funds flow).

Funds flow statement of ABC Ltd. Co. would appear as follows :

SOURCES OF FUND

	Rs. in lac
Funds from trading operation	3,850
Issue of shares at premium	2,000
Raising loan	2,300
	8,150

APPLICATION OF FUNDS

Purchase of fixed assets capital	1,500
Capital work in progress	3,000
Purchase of long term investments and loans	1,500
Payment of dividend	800
Payment of tax	1,500
	8,300

Application are highest man sources by Rs. 150 lacs. Thus working amount capital balance got reduced by the same amount.

CASH FLOW ANALYSIS

Cash flows are crucial to business decision. Cash is invested in the business and the rationality of such investment is evaluated taking into account the future cash flows it is expected to generate. The economic value of an asset is derived on the basis of its ability to generate future cash flows. The economic value of an asset is given by the present value of future cash flows expected to be derived from the asset.

Profit and cash flows from operations activities are not the same. Dividend decision is taken on the basis of profit, although it is to be paid in cash. Similarly, debt servicing capacity of a company is determined on the basis of cash flows from operations before interest. Ploughing back profit is a much talked about source of financing modernization, expansion and diversification. Unless retained profit is supported by cash, ploughing back is not possible. Thus cash flow analysis is an important basis for making several management decisions.

DIFFERENCE BETWEEN FUNDS FLOW AND CASH FLOW

Funds flow explains the reasons for changes in working capital whereas cash flows explains the reasons for changes in cash and cash equivalents.

In funds flow analysis, we have considered a concept funds from operations which do not reflect cash profit. To arrive at cash profit it is necessary to make adjustments for changes in current assets and current liabilities. Any increase in current assets reduces cash profit and any decrease. Increases cash profit. On the other hand, any increase in current liabilities increases cash profit and any decrease in current liabilities reduces cash profit. All other sources and applications of funds and cash flows are alike.

CLASSIFICATION OF CASH FLOW

Cash flow is classified into three broad categories

(a) **Cash flows from operating activities.** It is the net cash flows from revenue transactions arriving out of recurring and other operating activities.

(b) **Cash flows from investment activities.** Cash flows that represent cash transactions relating to investment in tangible and intangible fixed assets, long term investments and investments by way of long term loans and advances to others. They include interest and dividend received from investments.

(c) **Cash flows from financing activities.** Cash flows that represent raising of capital by way of issuing shares, debentures and raising long term loans and advances and repayment thereof. They include interest, dividend and redemption premium.

CASH FLOW STATEMENT

Various cash flows are put together in a cash flow statement. For example

Cash flow statement	**Rs. in lacs**
Cash flow from operating activities	(450)
Tax payment	(550)
Cash flow from investment activities	(1250)
Cash flow from financing activities	(1750)
Decrease in cash and cash equivalents	(50)

Thus, the cash flow statement explains the cash flow arising out of three major management function operations, investments and financing.

Cash flow statement is largely used for management decisions. However, there is a global trend in favour of inclusion of cash flow statement as a part of corporate financial statements. The SEBI has already issued a notification requiring listed comprises to include a cash flow statement in the annual report.

PROFIT PLANNING

The basic goal of any business — large or small is to earn profits. Profits determine the financial position, liquidity and solvency of a firm. Profit planning is, therefore, a vital part of business management.

Profit planning is the process of fore casting profits, formulating profit goals and policy and preparing budgets to maintain the desired level of activity and thereby to achieve the profit goals. Profit planning is based on the knowledge of various factors influencing profits and there inter-relationship. The main factors affecting profits are :

(i) **Selling price.** An increase in selling price tends to increase the profits and vice versa if the selling volume remains constant.

(ii) **Cost.** Increase in cost per unit tends to reduce price and vice versa.

(iii) **Volume.** It means the level of activity e.g. volume or value of production/sales.

(iv) **Product Mix.** Changes in the mix of products may also cause changes in profits.

A business firm can achieve its largest profit by varying one or more of the above variables.

Breakeven analysis is a widely used technique to study relationships between costs, price, sales volume and profits. It is a system of analysis which determines probable profit at any level of activity. It also determines the level of activity where total cost equals total sales revenue. Breakeven analysis is also known as cost volume profit analysis.

ROLE OF BREAKEVEN ANALYSIS IN PROFIT PLANNING

Breakeven analysis provides detailed information about the following things :

(a) The behavior of cost in relation to volume.

(b) Volume of production or sale, where the business will break even.

(c) Effect of variations in output on profits.

(d) Amount of profit for the projected sales volume.

(e) Production and sales volume required for a target level of profits.

(f) Effect of changes in costs and prices on profits.

Breakeven analysis helps in profit planning in following ways:

(a) It helps to determine changes in profits due to changes in costs, prices, volumes and product mix.

(b) It helps in executing profit targets by indicating production and sales levels required to achieve the desired profits.

(c) It helps in forecasting future profits with a fair degree of accuracy.

(d) It is useful in preparing flexible budgets by enabling management to predict profit over a wide range of volume.

(e) It assists management in evaluating profit performance of the company.

(f) It facilitates decision-making concerning installed capacity and its utilization.

(g) It helps in determining the amount of overhead costs to be charged at different levels of operations.

(h) It facilitates cost control by measuring operational efficiency of the plant.

11 SUPPORT TO SMALL SCALE INDUSTRIES

INSTITUTIONAL ASSISTANCE TO SSI's

Various institutions provide financial, training, law, export etc. assistance to Small Scale Industries.

Support at all India level is provided by

- Department of SSI (Ministry of Industries)
- Small Scale Industries Board
- Small Industries Development Organisation
- Specialised Institutions
- National Small Industries Corporation.

Support at state level is provided by

- State Directorate of Industries
- State Small Scale Industries Development Corporations
- Industrial Estates
- Technical Consultancy Organisations.

ALL THESE INSTITUTES ARE CREATED TO FACILITATE THE GROWTH OF SMALL SCALE SECTOR

Some of these institutes are discussed in detail

1. Small Scale Industries Board (SSIB)

SSIB was created in 1954 to advise on the programme and policies for the development of small scale sector. This board is also known as the Central Small Industries Board. The SSIB consists of 50 members including the representatives of the central and state governments, the Reserve Bank of India, the State Band of India and non-officials. The Union Industries Minister is the Chairman of the Board. The main work of SSIB are:

(a) To co-ordinate the activities of the National Small Industries Corporation and the Small Industries Service Institute.

(b) To offer advice on modifications or improvements for SSI in the country.

(c) The Board has adopted liberal terms of credit for small scale units. Bank credits to artisans, village and cottage industries is to be treated as composite term loan for equipment or working capital or both. Also the rate of interest for all term loans has been brought down to 16 percent.

2. Small Industries Development Organisation (SIDO)

SIDO is the apex level organisation set up for policy making, co-ordinating and monitoring agency for the development of SSI. It maintains close liaison with Govt., financial institutions and other agencies which are involved in the promotion and development of SSI. Development commissioner of small scale industries in the chief of the small industries development organisation. The SIDO functions though a network of 27 offices, 31 Small Industries Service Institutes (SISI), 37 extension centres, 3 product cum process development centres, 4 production cum testing centres and 4 regional testing centres.

The main function of SIDO are classified into three main categories

(i) Function relating to coordination

(a) Evolution of a national policy for the development of SSI.

(b) Coordination of the programme for the development of industrial estates.

(c) Maintaining liasion with the relevant Central Ministry, Planning Commission, State Governments, Financial Institutions etc.

(ii) Functions relating to industrial development

(a) Securing items reserved for production by SSI.

(b) Rendering support for the development of ancillaries.

(c) Preparing model schemes, project reports and other technical literature for prospective entrepreneurs.

(iii) Functions relating to extension services

(a) Provision for consultancy and training to strengthen the competitiveness of SSI.

(b) Provision for marketing assistance to SSI to market there products.

(c) Provision for economic investigation and information services to SSI.

3. National Small Industries Corporation (NSIC)

It was set up in 1955 as a public undertaking. It is engaged in promoting and developing SSI in the country. Its main work is supply of machineries on hire purchase basis. The main functions are

(i) Supplying machinery on hire purchase basis.

(ii) Procuring government orders for SSI.

(iii) Developing SSI as ancillaries to large industries.

(iv) Arranging the marketing of products of SSI and promoting exports.

(v) Importing and distributing scarce raw materials, components and parts among actual users in small scale sector.

(vi) Undertaking the construction of industrial estates.

4. Industrial Estates (I.E.)

It is yet another measure to promote industrialization in the country.

DEFINITION

An industrial estate is a group of factories, constructed on an economic scale in suitable sites with facilities of water, transport, electricity, bank, hospital etc. and provided with special arrangements for technical guidance and common service facilities.

Thus an industrial estate is a place where the required facilities and factory accommodation are provided by the government to the entrepreneurs to establish their industries there.

OBJECTIVES OF INDUSTRIES ESTATES

(a) To provide infrastructure and accommodation facilities to the entrepreneurs.

(b) To encourage the development of SSI in the country.

(c) To decentralize industries to the rural and backward areas.

(d) To encourage ancillarisation in surrounding major industrial units.

(e) To develop entrepreneurship by creating a congerial climate to run the industries in these estates/areas etc.

INDUSTRIES ESTATES IN INDIA

1. The idea of establishing industries estate was first adopted in India by the Small Scale Industries Board (SSIB) in Jan. 1955.
2. So first industries estate in India was set up at Rajkot in Gujarat in Sept. 1955.
3. By now the number of industrial estates is more than 650.

TYPES OF INDUSTRIES ESTATES

1. On the basis of function
   (i) General type I.E.
   (ii) Special type I.E.
2. On the basis of organisational set up
   (i) Govt. Industrial Estate

(ii) Pvt. Industrial Estate
(iii) Co-operative Industries estate
(iv) Municipal Industrial Estate

3. On the basis of other variants
   (i) Ancillary Industrial Estate (Ancillary to main industries)
   (ii) Functional Industrial Estate (Manufacturing some product)
   (iii) The workshop bay (Repair/services industries)

REASONS FOR POOR PERFORMANCE OF INDUSTRIES ESTATES

1. Lack of essential infrastructure such as a roads, power water etc.
2. Lack of common facilities such as tool room, testing etc.
3. Lack of realistic survey prior to the establishment of the estate
4. Lack of a clear idea about the relevance of products to the area.
5. Lack of local involvement and active participation in the programme.

FACTORS ESSENTIAL FOR SUCCESSFUL INDUSTRIAL ESTATE

1. Existence of large number of small firms in appropriate industrial sector.
2. Entrepreneurs willing and able to take advantage of the facilities offered by the industrial estate.
3. A nucleus of skilled workers.
4. Govt. agencies with skills and funds to plan and administer the plan.
5. Financial institutions willing to give credit to the units.
6. Availability of adequate infrastructure in terms of water, electricity and transport.

5. Specialised Institutions

1. **Central Institute of Tool Design, Hyderabad.** The Central Govt. set up the institute in 1968 with the help of UNDP and ILO to help SSI by importing specialised training to the personal working in the design and manufacture of tools, dies, moulds etc. The other functions performed by it are:
   (a) To offer consultancy and advisory services and assistance in the design and development of tools.
   (b) To suggest proper measures to improve the standard of tools, tooling elements, dies etc.
   (c) To offer the needed tool room facility.

   A governing council which consists of representatives of the Govt. and industry is constituted to look after the management of the institute. The governing council is headed by the Development Commissioner (SSI).

2. **National Institute of Entrepreneurship and Small Business Development (NIESBUD).** It is an apex national level institute of its kind set up at New Delhi in 1983. Its main functions are to co-ordinate research and training in entrepreneurship development and to impart specialised training to various categories of entrepreneurs. Besides, it also serves as a farum for interaction and exchange of views between various agencies engaged in activities relating to entrepreneurial development.
3. **National Institute of Small Industries Extension Training (NISIET), Hyderabad.** This institute was set up is 1956 to develop the required manpower for running small scale industries in the country. Its main functions are—
   (a) To impart training to the persons engaged in SSI.
   (b) To undertake research studies relating to development of SSI.
   (c) To enter into agreements relating to consultancy services both with national and international organisation to provide consultancy services to small industries in country.

   The institute conducts courses in business management for the benefit of the entrepreneurs and semi-managerial personnels of SSI.

12 TAXATION BENEFITS TO SMALL SCALE INDUSTRIES

Small scale industries need helping hand to grow and succeed. The Govt. offers them various tax benefits to lend a supporting hand to SSI.

In the beginning, small industries have to incur more expenses, but the returns are either nil or nominal. Therefore, they need to be provided assistance to enable them to survive. The Govt. has come forward with various benefits to offer to small scale industries in the country. The Govt. either exempts them from tax or provides them concession in tax. This helps small industries accumulate capital, on the one hand and plough back profits in business on the other. The various tax benefits available to SSI are—

1. Tax holiday

Under section 80J of the Income Tax Act 1961, new industrial undertakings, including small scale industries, are exempted from the payment of income-tax on their profits subject to a maximum of 6% per annum of main capital employed. This exemption in tax is allowed for a period of five years from the commencement of production. A SSI has to satisfy the following two conditions to avail of this tax exemption facility.

(i) The unit should not have been formed by the splitting or reconstitution of an existing unit.

(ii) The unit should not employ 10 or more workers in a manufacturing. process with power or at least 20 workers without power.

2. Depreciation

Under section 32 of the Income Tax Act, 1961, a SSI is entitled to a deduction on depreciation account on block of assets at the prescribed rate. In the case of SSI, deduction from the actual cost of plant and machinery is allowed subject to a maximum of Rs. 20 lakhs. A SSI should satisfy the following conditions before it becomes eligible for deduction in depreciation.

(i) The assets should be owned by the assessee.

(ii) The assets must actually be used for the purpose of the assessee's business or profession.

(iii) Depreciation allowance or deduction is allowed only on fixed assets i.e., building, machinery, plant and furniture.

3. Rehabilitation allowance

A rehabilitation allowance is granted to small scale industry under section 33-B of the Income Tax Act, 1961 whose business is discontinued on account of following reasons—

(i) Flood, typhoon, hurricanes cyclone, earthquakes etc.

(ii) Riot or civil disturbance.

(iii) Accidental fire or explosion.

(iv) Action takes by an enemy etc.

The rehabilitation allowance should be used for business purposes within three years of unit's re-establishment, reconstruction.

4. Investment allowance

This was introduced in 1976 to replace the initial depreciation allowance. The investment allowance under section 31 A of the Income Tax Act 1961, is allowed at the rate of 25% of the cost of acquisition of new plant or machinery installed.

A SSI can avail of investment allowance provided it has put to use machinery or plant either in the year of installation or in the following year failing which the benefit will be forfeited.

5. Expenditure an acquisition of patents and copyrights

Under section 35 A of the Income Tax Act, 1961, any expenditure of a capital nature incurred in acquiring a patent and copyright by a SSI is deductible from its income. The expenditure can be deduced in 14 equal installments beginning with the previous year in which the expenditure was incurred in acquiring patents and copyrights for the units.

6. Tax concessions to SSI in rural areas

Under section 80-HHA in the Income Tax Act 1961, the tax payers are entitled to a deduction of 20% of the profits and gains derived by running SSI in rural areas. The deduction is allowed for a period of 10 years from the year of commencement of manufacturing activity after 30th Sept. 1977. This benefit is not allowed to SSI engaged in mining activities. The SSI can avail this tax deduction only if following conditions are satisfied.

(i) The SSI is not formed by splitting or reconstruction of a business already in existence.

(ii) It is not formed by transfer to a new business of machinery or plant previously used for any purpose.

(iii) The accounts of the unit are audited by a chartered accountant.

(iv) It employs 10 or more workers in manufacturing process carried on with power or 20 or more workers in a manufacturing process carried on without power.

(v) The unit doesn't claim a simultaneous deduction under section 80-HH of the Income Tax Act 1961.

7. Tax concessions to SSI in backward areas

In 1970-71, the Planning Commission of India declared 247 districts as backward areas with a view to provide them special incentives and concessions for establishment of industries in them. The SSI newly established in those areas are entitled to a deduction of 20% of main profits and gains from these gross total income. This deduction is allowed for a period of 10 years beginning with the year of commencement of production.

However if a SSI has already been established in a non-backward area and later shifts to a backward area, the unit will be allowed this deduction on the profits earned from the unit after shifting in the backward area for period of 10 years. This tax benefit is not allowed to the SSI engaged in mining activites. The unit has to satisfy following conditions:

(i) It is established on or after 31st Dec. 1970.

(ii) It employs atleast 10 workers in a manufacturing process with the aid of power or at least 20 workers in a manufacturing process without the aid of power.

8. MODVAT and SSI (MODVAT: Modified Value Added tax)

This scheme intends to greatly and gradually expand its horizon to set off excise and other countervailing duties paid on various inputs of final product. This aims at coming closer to a generalised get-off excise taxation on inputs. For this, the basic approach to be followed is to move towards the extension of ongoing system of proforma credit to all excisable commodities. A few sector/product like textile products, petroleum and tobacco have been left for this purpose.

13 LAWS FOR SMALL SCALE INDUSTRIES

Central and State Govt. have made several laws to regulate, promote and protect the growth of SSI in India. Some of these laws are summarized as following:

1. Workman's Compensation Act, 1923
2. Trade Union Act, 1926
3. Provident Funds Act, 1952
4. ESI Act, 1948
5. Payment of Bonus Act, 1965
6. Payment of Gratuity Act, 1972
7. Industrial Disputes Act, 1947
8. Industrial Employment (Standing Orders) Act, 1946.

1. The Workmen's Compensation Act, 1923

1. The wage limit for coverage has been raised from Rs. 400 to Rs 500.
2. A workman is entitled to compensation within two years from the date, the symptoms of any disease develop after leaning employment.
3. Any person employed on monthly wages upto Rs. 1,000 is covered under this act.

Privileges induced in wages

1. Free accommodation
2. Maternity benefit
3. DA
4. Overtime
5. Benefits in form of food, clothing, concession etc.

These are not wages

1. T.A
2. Contribution of employer towards pension or P.F.

COMPENSATION

1. Compensation in case of death = 40% of monthly wages × relevant factor or 24,000 whichever is more

2. Compensation in case of permanent disablement (Total) = 50% of monthly wages × relevant factor or 24,000 whichever is more.
3. Compensation is case of permanent (partial) disablement — Percent of loss in earning capacity as given in part II schedule I of act.
4. Compensation in case of temp. disablement total or partial — Recurring half monthly payment of the sum equivalent to 25% of monthly wages till the period of disablement or 5 years whichever is short.

2. Provident Funds Act, 1952

This Act is not applicable to organisation having less man 50 persons.

Contribution to scheme = 12% of (Basic wages + D.A. + cash value of food concession + retaining allowance as member employee's contribution) = an equivalent of 12% will be employer's contribution.

On this contribution, there will be a compound interest added at the rate of 13% every year.

3. ESI Act, 1948

This act applies to employees whose wages (Basic + VDA + HRA, CCA, P.P. and OSA) including overtime wages are Rs. 6500 or less per month.

It includes all permanent, temporary, casual contract workers etc. The employer and employee contributes in the scheme. 1.75% of employee's wages are employee contribution and 4.75% of employee's wages as employer's contribution are to be deposited by the employer in ESIC account in treasury with 20 days of completion of each wage period.

BENEFITS

1. **Medical benefits**
2. **Sickness benefits**. This can be availed for a max. Period of 8 weeks in a year.
3. **Maternity benefit**. 4½ months.
4. **Disablement benefit**
5. **Dependent's benefit**. Deceased person's sons and daughters get pension till age 18 and wife-lifelong or till she remarries.
6. **Occupational disease benefit.**

4. Payment of Bonus Act, 1965

1. Act will apply to every organisation in which 20 or more workers are employed.
2. Every employee is eligible for bonus unless he has worked for not less than 30 days.
3. **Payment of minimum bonus.** 8.33% of salary earned by the employee during the accounting year or Rs. 100/- whichever is higher.

4. **Payment of maximum bonus**. Where allocable surplus exceeds the amount of minimum bonus payable, the employer shall pay proportionately to the salary/ wages earned by employees, subject to maximum of 20% of such salary or wages.
5. **Eligibility**. Any employee who is getting a salary/wage up to Rs. 3,500/- per month shall be entitled for payment of bonus under this act, but calculations for bonus payment shall be made on maximum Rs. 2500/- only. Bonus will be paid on basic, DA etc. and not on HRA.
6. **Time limit.** Bonus shall be paid within a period of 8 months from the date of closing of accounting year.

5. Payment of Gratuity Act, 1972

This act apply to every factory having 10 or more persons i.e. employees.

1. **Payment.** Gratuity shall be payable to as employee on termination of service after rendering continuous service for not less than 5 years on retirement, resignation etc.

   In case of death completion of 5 years continuous service is not necessary.
2. **Amount.** The amount of gratuity shall not exceed 20 months wages i.e., not more than Rs. 1,00,000/-.
3. **Formula for calculation of gratuity**

$$\text{Gratuity} = \frac{\text{Last drawn pay} \times 15 \text{ days} \times \text{No. of years of service}}{26}$$

6. Industrial Disputes Act, 1947

Retrenchment. Employee is paid 15 days average pay for every completed year of continuous service.

Lay off. 50% of total of basic wages and D.A. for all days during which he is laid off.

AUTHORITIES IN THIS ACT

1. **Section 3. Works committee.** 100 or more employees. Their decision coarries weight but is not concluctive.
2. **Section 4. Conciliation officer.** Duty is of mediating and promoting the settlement of industrial disputes.
3. **Section 5. Boards of conciliation.** It consists of a chairman and 2 or 4 other members. Chairman is an independent person (conciliation).
4. **Section 6. Court of enquiry.** Consists of one or more independent persons and out of which one is chairman. Report will be made within 6 month from the commencement of inquiry (investigation).

5. **Section 7. Labour Court.** Schedule I cases. It consists of one person only to be appointed by appropriate government, who will be the presiding officer of the labour court (The officer should be judge of a High Court/or for minimum 3 years District Judge/or for minimum 2 years officer/Chairman of Tribunal etc.).
6. **Section 7A. Industrial tribunal.** Scheduls II and III cases. It consists of one person only. (Officer should be judge of High Court/or minimum 3 years District Judge/minimum 2 years Chairman of Tribunal).
7. **Section 7B. National tribunal. (Adjudication)** Consists of one person only.

Compensations for

(a) **Closer.** Not exceed his average pay for 3 months.

(b) **Lay-off.** Paid for all days during which laid-off except for weekly holidays and compensation shall be equal to 50% of the total basic wages and D.A. (after 45 days no payment).

(c) **Retrenchment.** Worker is given 3 months notice in writing indicating the reasons for retrenchment.

7. The Industrial Employment (Standing orders) Act 1946.

This act applies to organisation having more than 100 employees.

1. The employer of every industrial establishment to which this act applies is required to frame a draft standing orders and to submit them to the certifying officer, who is generally, the labour commissioner for certification.
2. **Procedure for certification.** The employer should submit to the certifying officer 5 copies of the draft standing orders proposed to be adopted by him together with the prescribed particulars of workman employed and Trade Union etc. Any objections can be submitted by the worker within 14 days after the certifying officer has forwarded a copy thereof to the Trade Union of standing orders. The certifying officer or appellate authoring shall have the power to adjudicate upon the fairness of the provision of the standing order.
3. **Date of operation.** Standing orders will, unless an appeal is preferred, come into operation on the expiry of 30 days from the date on which the copies of the same are sent.
4. **Modification in orders.** Only after 6 months or as per agreement between employer and employee.
5. **Payment of subsistence**

   (a) At the rate of 50% of wages from date of suspension till 90 days.

   (b) At rate of 75% of wages for the remaining period of suspension if the delay in completion of disciplinary proceedings against such workman is not directly attributable to the conduct of such workman.

QUESTION BANK OF ENTREPRENEURSHIP DEVELOPMENT PROGRAMME

1. Explain the concept of entrepreneur? How does an entrepreneur differ from a manager?
2. "Entrepreneurs are made not born". Comment.
3. Explain the distinguishing characteristics of a successful entrepreneur.
4. "Entrepreneurship does not emerge spontaneously". Discuss.
6. Discuss the role of entrepreneurs in the economic development of a country.
6. What are the problems faced by entrepreneur.
7. "Developing countries need imitative rather than innovative entrepreneurs". Comment.
8. "Entrepreneurs and entrepreneurship are the catalysts in the process of economic development of a country". Explain.
9. Explain in detail the factors which help in the development of entrepreneurship.
10. Explain the concept of entrepreneurs, intrapreneur and entrepreneurship.
11. Differentiate between entrepreneurs and intrapreneurs.
12. Define entrepreneurs and explain their characteristics and explain their different types.
13. "Innovation is the hallmark of entrepreneurship". Explain.
14. Write short notes on.
    (a) Intrapreneurs
    (b) Innovative entrepreneurs
    (c) Main functions of entrepreneurs
    (d) Immitative entrepreneurs.
15. What is the importance of SSI in the development of economy?
16. How is government policy beneficial for the development of SSI? Justify your answers with example.

17. Define SSI. What are its chief characteristics?
18. What is the rationale behind the development of SSI in India?
19. "SSI serves as a seedbed of entrepreneurship development". Explain.
20. Appreciate the role of SSI in the development of national economy.
21. Discuss the need for policy support to SSI.
22. Write a note on causes of sickness in SSI.
23. Differentiate between SSI and ancillary units.
24. Explain in short the steps in starting a SSI.
25. What is meant by project formulation? Explain.
26. How will you judge the feasibility of a new project? Explain the various feaibility techniques.
27. Describe the need and significance of preparing a project report.
28. "Project evaluation is a comprehensive task". Discuss.
29. Write short notes on
    (a) Risk analysis
    (b) Demand analysis
    (c) Technical feasibility
    (d) Market survey
    (e) Economic viability
    (f) Financial feasibility
30. What is "Project formulation"? How is it important in the starting of a new project?
31. Explain the purpose of connducting a techno economic study before launching a project.
32. Mention the various sources of deriving business idea and explain project selection.
33. What is a project report? Explain the contents of a project report.
34. What do you mean by project appraisal.
35. What are the different forms of business ownership? Which one of these would you prefer in case of a small enterprise and why?
36. Differentiate between partnership firm and Pvt. Ltd. Co.
37. Discuss the merits and demerits of partnership as a form of business organisation.
38. A SSI can be started either as sole proprietorship or as a partnership. Discuss the relative merits of these forms of ownerships.

39. "Corporate form of business is superior to proprietary or partnership form of ownership". Explain with reference to merits and demerits of each.
40. What factors decide location of an industry.
41. What are the various types of plant layout.
42. Explain the benefits of a good plant layout.
43. Discuss the factors which affect plant layout decision.
44. Describe the meaning and significance of plant location.
45. What is production control? What are the main functioins involved in it?
46. What do you mean by production/manufacturing planing? What steps are involved in it?
47. What is appropriate technology for small business? How will you decide such technology?
48. Define quality control. How can quality be controlled in small firms.
49. Discuss the concept of TQC and explain its salient features.
50. Describe the various techniques of quality control.
51. Write short notes on
    (a) Localional analysis
    (b) Plant layout
    (c) SQC
    (d) TQM
    (e) Control charts
    (f) Routing and scheduling in a plant.
52. What is the meaning and functions of inventory control?
53. Explain EOQ model.
54. Illustrate the operation of continuous review and periodic review systems.
55. Inventory management helps to minimise cash outlays and the success of a small firm depends on its control. "Elucidate."
56. Write short notes on
    (a) EOQ model
    (b) ABC analysis
    (c) Inventory systems (continuous and periodic)
    (d) Inventory costs.
57. Discuss in brief the procedure which a SSI should follow for buying raw materials.
58. Discuss the nature and objectives of purchase function in a SSI.

59. What are the various fringe benefits available to an employee? Why are they necessary?

60. "Globalization has thrown up new challenges for IR manager. Comment.

61. Why do grievances arise in an industry?

62. What are the various wage payment and incentive methods being used by the organisations.

63. Suggest suitable steps to handle grievances successfully.

64. Explain the machinery for the settlement of industrial disputes (judicial and non- judicial).

65. Bring out clearly the nature, scope and importance of I.R. in the context of present day industrial setup.

66. Explain the parties to I.R. Why do disputes arise?

67. Write short notes on

(a) Step ladder grievance procedure

(b) Standing orders

(c) Essentials of good grievance procedure

(d) Nature of grievances.

68. How does performance is appraised?

69. "Motivation and leadership is necessary for the success of any SSI/business firm". Comment.

70. Explain the problems of marketing is SSI in India?

71. "Distribution channel brings products from produces to consumes". Explain. What considerations should be kept in mind while selecting a suitable channel of distribution?

72. Write short notes on

(a) Marketing mix

(b) Market segmentation

(c) Advertising methods

(d) Branding

(e) Distribution channel

(f) Pricing policies.

73. What are the objectives of pricing? Explain the main pricing policies.

74. "The success of small enterprise greatly depends upon their ability in marketing of their products". In the light of this statement bring out the marketing problems and activities of SSI.

75. "Advertising is wasteful". Do you agree? Give reasons in support of your answer.
76. Define industrial estates. What are their objectives? How do they assist SSI?
77. Write notes on
    (a) SSIB
    (b) Industrial estates
    (c) SSIDC
    (d) Specialised institutes
    (e) SIDO
    (f) Tax holiday
    (g) MODVAT
    (h) Rehabilitation allowance
    (i) Depreciation allowance.
78. Explain tax benefits available to SSI.
79. Give a review of various industrial policy resolutions with reference to SSI.
80. What are the salient features of eight five year industrial policy w.r.t. SSI?
81. Describe the various policies and programmes of Govt. for improving the growth of SSI in the country.
82. Distinguish between journal and ledger. How does a trial balance help in preparation of final accounts?
83. How can a small scale unit maintain its accounts?
84. Write short notes on
    (a) Working capital
    (b) Fixed capital
    (c) Operating cycle
    (d) Cash flow analysis
    (*e*) Financial ratio analysis
    (f) Funds flow analysis
    (g) Balance sheet
    (h) Profit planning and programming.
85. What are the various sources of capital available to small scale businessman for raising capital?
86. Explain the role and support of SBI and SIDBI in financial working area of SSI.
87. Discuss the factors that influence the working capital requirements of a firm.
88. Explain the exemptions from central sales tax, 1956?

89. What benefits are available to injured workmen under the Workmen's Compensation Act, 1923?
90. Explain the exemptions offered to SSI in income tax.
91. "Does every problem require a decision"? Describe the process involved in decision making.
92. Discuss the special tax benefits available to SSI operating in rural and economically backward areas.
93. Write a note on salient features of New Small Enterprise Policy, 1991.
94. What is 'cost of capital'? Underline the importance and relevance of cost of capital approach in project planning and control.
95. "For the industrial development of India, both SSI and LSI need to develop as mutually supportive and complementary to each other". Discuss.

INDEX

Q

R

S

T

V

W

Z